# Pharmaceutical Process Engineering

## DRUGS AND THE PHARMACEUTICAL SCIENCES

## DRUGS AND THE PHARMACEUTICAL SCIENCES

A Series of Textbooks and Monographs

1. Pharmacokinetics, *Milo Gibaldi and Donald Perrier*
2. Good Manufacturing Practices for Pharmaceuticals: A Plan for Total Quality Control, *Sidney H. Willig, Murray M. Tuckerman, and William S. Hitchings IV*
3. Microencapsulation, *edited by J. R. Nixon*
4. Drug Metabolism: Chemical and Biochemical Aspects, *Bernard Testa and Peter Jenner*
5. New Drugs: Discovery and Development, *edited by Alan A. Rubin*
6. Sustained and Controlled Release Drug Delivery Systems, *edited by Joseph R. Robinson*
7. Modern Pharmaceutics, *edited by Gilbert S. Banker and Christopher T. Rhodes*
8. Prescription Drugs in Short Supply: Case Histories, *Michael A. Schwartz*
9. Activated Charcoal: Antidotal and Other Medical Uses, *David O. Cooney*
10. Concepts in Drug Metabolism (in two parts), *edited by Peter Jenner and Bernard Testa*
11. Pharmaceutical Analysis: Modern Methods (in two parts), *edited by James W. Munson*
12. Techniques of Solubilization of Drugs, *edited by Samuel H. Yalkowsky*
13. Orphan Drugs, *edited by Fred E. Karch*
14. Novel Drug Delivery Systems: Fundamentals, Developmental Concepts, Biomedical Assessments, *Yie W. Chien*
15. Pharmacokinetics: Second Edition, Revised and Expanded, *Milo Gibaldi and Donald Perrier*
16. Good Manufacturing Practices for Pharmaceuticals: A Plan for Total Quality Control, Second Edition, Revised and Expanded, *Sidney H. Willig, Murray M. Tuckerman, and William S. Hitchings IV*
17. Formulation of Veterinary Dosage Forms, *edited by Jack Blodinger*
18. Dermatological Formulations: Percutaneous Absorption, *Brian W. Barry*
19. The Clinical Research Process in the Pharmaceutical Industry, *edited by Gary M. Matoren*
20. Microencapsulation and Related Drug Processes, *Patrick B. Deasy*
21. Drugs and Nutrients: The Interactive Effects, *edited by Daphne A. Roe and T. Colin Campbell*
22. Biotechnology of Industrial Antibiotics, *Erick J. Vandamme*

23. Pharmaceutical Process Validation, *edited by Bernard T. Loftus and Robert A. Nash*
24. Anticancer and Interferon Agents: Synthesis and Properties, *edited by Raphael M. Ottenbrite and George B. Butler*
25. Pharmaceutical Statistics: Practical and Clinical Applications, *Sanford Bolton*
26. Drug Dynamics for Analytical, Clinical, and Biological Chemists, *Benjamin J. Gudzinowicz, Burrows T. Younkin, Jr., and Michael J. Gudzinowicz*
27. Modern Analysis of Antibiotics, *edited by Adjoran Aszalos*
28. Solubility and Related Properties, *Kenneth C. James*
29. Controlled Drug Delivery: Fundamentals and Applications, Second Edition, Revised and Expanded, *edited by Joseph R. Robinson and Vincent H. Lee*
30. New Drug Approval Process: Clinical and Regulatory Management, *edited by Richard A. Guarino*
31. Transdermal Controlled Systemic Medications, *edited by Yie W. Chien*
32. Drug Delivery Devices: Fundamentals and Applications, *edited by Praveen Tyle*
33. Pharmacokinetics: Regulatory • Industrial • Academic Perspectives, *edited by Peter G. Welling and Francis L. S. Tse*
34. Clinical Drug Trials and Tribulations, *edited by Allen E. Cato*
35. Transdermal Drug Delivery: Developmental Issues and Research Initiatives, *edited by Jonathan Hadgraft and Richard H. Guy*
36. Aqueous Polymeric Coatings for Pharmaceutical Dosage Forms, *edited by James W. McGinity*
37. Pharmaceutical Pelletization Technology, *edited by Isaac Ghebre-Sellassie*
38. Good Laboratory Practice Regulations, *edited by Allen F. Hirsch*
39. Nasal Systemic Drug Delivery, *Yie W. Chien, Kenneth S. E. Su, and Shyi-Feu Chang*
40. Modern Pharmaceutics: Second Edition, Revised and Expanded, *edited by Gilbert S. Banker and Christopher T. Rhodes*
41. Specialized Drug Delivery Systems: Manufacturing and Production Technology, *edited by Praveen Tyle*
42. Topical Drug Delivery Formulations, *edited by David W. Osborne and Anton H. Amann*
43. Drug Stability: Principles and Practices, *Jens T. Carstensen*
44. Pharmaceutical Statistics: Practical and Clinical Applications, Second Edition, Revised and Expanded, *Sanford Bolton*
45. Biodegradable Polymers as Drug Delivery Systems, *edited by Mark Chasin and Robert Langer*
46. Preclinical Drug Disposition: A Laboratory Handbook, *Francis L. S. Tse and James J. Jaffe*
47. HPLC in the Pharmaceutical Industry, *edited by Godwin W. Fong and Stanley K. Lam*
48. Pharmaceutical Bioequivalence, *edited by Peter G. Welling, Francis L. S. Tse, and Shrikant V. Dinghe*

49. Pharmaceutical Dissolution Testing, *Umesh V. Banakar*
50. Novel Drug Delivery Systems: Second Edition, Revised and Expanded, *Yie W. Chien*
51. Managing the Clinical Drug Development Process, *David M. Cocchetto and Ronald V. Nardi*
52. Good Manufacturing Practices for Pharmaceuticals: A Plan for Total Quality Control, Third Edition, *edited by Sidney H. Willig and James R. Stoker*
53. Prodrugs: Topical and Ocular Drug Delivery, *edited by Kenneth B. Sloan*
54. Pharmaceutical Inhalation Aerosol Technology, *edited by Anthony J. Hickey*
55. Radiopharmaceuticals: Chemistry and Pharmacology, *edited by Adrian D. Nunn*
56. New Drug Approval Process: Second Edition, Revised and Expanded, *edited by Richard A. Guarino*
57. Pharmaceutical Process Validation: Second Edition, Revised and Expanded, *edited by Ira R. Berry and Robert A. Nash*
58. Ophthalmic Drug Delivery Systems, *edited by Ashim K. Mitra*
59. Pharmaceutical Skin Penetration Enhancement, *edited by Kenneth A. Walters and Jonathan Hadgraft*
60. Colonic Drug Absorption and Metabolism, *edited by Peter R. Bieck*
61. Pharmaceutical Particulate Carriers: Therapeutic Applications, *edited by Alain Rolland*
62. Drug Permeation Enhancement: Theory and Applications, *edited by Dean S. Hsieh*
63. Glycopeptide Antibiotics, *edited by Ramakrishnan Nagarajan*
64. Achieving Sterility in Medical and Pharmaceutical Products, *Nigel A. Halls*
65. Multiparticulate Oral Drug Delivery, *edited by Isaac Ghebre-Sellassie*
66. Colloidal Drug Delivery Systems, *edited by Jörg Kreuter*
67. Pharmacokinetics: Regulatory • Industrial • Academic Perspectives, Second Edition, *edited by Peter G. Welling and Francis L. S. Tse*
68. Drug Stability: Principles and Practices, Second Edition, Revised and Expanded, *Jens T. Carstensen*
69. Good Laboratory Practice Regulations: Second Edition, Revised and Expanded, *edited by Sandy Weinberg*
70. Physical Characterization of Pharmaceutical Solids, *edited by Harry G. Brittain*
71. Pharmaceutical Powder Compaction Technology, *edited by Göran Alderborn and Christer Nyström*
72. Modern Pharmaceutics: Third Edition, Revised and Expanded, *edited by Gilbert S. Banker and Christopher T. Rhodes*
73. Microencapsulation: Methods and Industrial Applications, *edited by Simon Benita*
74. Oral Mucosal Drug Delivery, *edited by Michael J. Rathbone*
75. Clinical Research in Pharmaceutical Development, *edited by Barry Bleidt and Michael Montagne*

76. The Drug Development Process: Increasing Efficiency and Cost Effectiveness, *edited by Peter G. Welling, Louis Lasagna, and Umesh V. Banakar*
77. Microparticulate Systems for the Delivery of Proteins and Vaccines, *edited by Smadar Cohen and Howard Bernstein*
78. Good Manufacturing Practices for Pharmaceuticals: A Plan for Total Quality Control, Fourth Edition, Revised and Expanded, *Sidney H. Willig and James R. Stoker*
79. Aqueous Polymeric Coatings for Pharmaceutical Dosage Forms: Second Edition, Revised and Expanded, *edited by James W. McGinity*
80. Pharmaceutical Statistics: Practical and Clinical Applications, Third Edition, *Sanford Bolton*
81. Handbook of Pharmaceutical Granulation Technology, *edited by Dilip M. Parikh*
82. Biotechnology of Antibiotics: Second Edition, Revised and Expanded, *edited by William R. Strohl*
83. Mechanisms of Transdermal Drug Delivery, *edited by Russell O. Potts and Richard H. Guy*
84. Pharmaceutical Enzymes, *edited by Albert Lauwers and Simon Scharpé*
85. Development of Biopharmaceutical Parenteral Dosage Forms, *edited by John A. Bontempo*
86. Pharmaceutical Project Management, *edited by Tony Kennedy*
87. Drug Products for Clinical Trials: An International Guide to Formulation • Production • Quality Control, *edited by Donald C. Monkhouse and Christopher T. Rhodes*
88. Development and Formulation of Veterinary Dosage Forms: Second Edition, Revised and Expanded, *edited by Gregory E. Hardee and J. Desmond Baggot*
89. Receptor-Based Drug Design, *edited by Paul Leff*
90. Automation and Validation of Information in Pharmaceutical Processing, *edited by Joseph F. deSpautz*
91. Dermal Absorption and Toxicity Assessment, *edited by Michael S. Roberts and Kenneth A. Walters*
92. Pharmaceutical Experimental Design, *Gareth A. Lewis, Didier Mathieu, and Roger Phan-Tan-Luu*
93. Preparing for FDA Pre-Approval Inspections, *edited by Martin D. Hynes III*
94. Pharmaceutical Excipients: Characterization by IR, Raman, and NMR Spectroscopy, *David E. Bugay and W. Paul Findlay*
95. Polymorphism in Pharmaceutical Solids, *edited by Harry G. Brittain*
96. Freeze-Drying/Lyophilization of Pharmaceutical and Biological Products, *edited by Louis Rey and Joan C. May*
97. Percutaneous Absorption: Drugs–Cosmetics–Mechanisms–Methodology, Third Edition, Revised and Expanded, *edited by Robert L. Bronaugh and Howard I. Maibach*

98. Bioadhesive Drug Delivery Systems: Fundamentals, Novel Approaches, and Development, *edited by Edith Mathiowitz, Donald E. Chickering III, and Claus-Michael Lehr*
99. Protein Formulation and Delivery, *edited by Eugene J. McNally*
100. New Drug Approval Process: Third Edition, The Global Challenge, *edited by Richard A. Guarino*
101. Peptide and Protein Drug Analysis, *edited by Ronald E. Reid*
102. Transport Processes in Pharmaceutical Systems, *edited by Gordon L. Amidon, Ping I. Lee, and Elizabeth M. Topp*
103. Excipient Toxicity and Safety, *edited by Myra L. Weiner and Lois A. Kotkoskie*
104. The Clinical Audit in Pharmaceutical Development, *edited by Michael R. Hamrell*
105. Pharmaceutical Emulsions and Suspensions, *edited by Francoise Nielloud and Gilberte Marti-Mestres*
106. Oral Drug Absorption: Prediction and Assessment, *edited by Jennifer B. Dressman and Hans Lennernäs*
107. Drug Stability: Principles and Practices, Third Edition, Revised and Expanded, *edited by Jens T. Carstensen and C. T. Rhodes*
108. Containment in the Pharmaceutical Industry, *edited by James P. Wood*
109. Good Manufacturing Practices for Pharmaceuticals: A Plan for Total Quality Control from Manufacturer to Consumer, Fifth Edition, Revised and Expanded, *Sidney H. Willig*
110. Advanced Pharmaceutical Solids, *Jens T. Carstensen*
111. Endotoxins: Pyrogens, LAL Testing, and Depyrogenation, Second Edition, Revised and Expanded, *Kevin L. Williams*
112. Pharmaceutical Process Engineering, *Anthony J. Hickey and David Ganderton*

**ADDITIONAL VOLUMES IN PREPARATION**

Handbook of Pharmaceutical Analysis, *edited by Lena Ohannesian and Anthony J. Streeter*

Pharmacogenomics, *edited by Werner Kalow, Urs A. Meyer, and Rachel Tyndale*

Drug–Drug Interactions, *David Rodrigues*

Handbook of Drug Screening, *edited by Ramakrishna Seethala and Prabhavathi Fernandes*

Drug Targeting Technology: A Critical Analysis of Physical • Chemical • Biological Methods, *edited by Hans Schreier*

# Pharmaceutical Process Engineering


Anthony J. Hickey

*University of North Carolina*
*Chapel Hill, North Carolina*

David Ganderton

*Vectura Limited*
*Bath, United Kingdom*


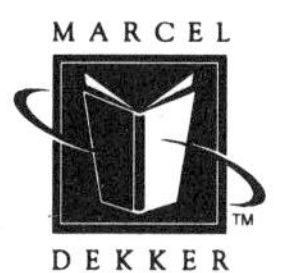



MARCEL DEKKER, INC. NEW YORK • BASEL

**ISBN: 0-8247-0298-0**

This book is printed on acid-free paper.

**Headquarters**
Marcel Dekker, Inc.
270 Madison Avenue, New York, NY 10016
tel: 212-696-9000; fax: 212-685-4540

**Eastern Hemisphere Distribution**
Marcel Dekker AG
Hutgasse 4, Postfach 812, CH-4001 Basel, Switzerland
tel: 41-61-261-8482; fax: 41-61-261-8896

**World Wide Web**
http://www.dekker.com

The publisher offers discounts on this book when ordered in bulk quantities. For more information, write to Special Sales/Professional Marketing at the headquarters address above.



Current printing (last digit):
10 9 8 7 6 5 4 3 2 1

**PRINTED IN THE UNITED STATES OF AMERICA**

# Preface

Early in my professional life I was introduced to David Ganderton's excellent text *Unit Processes in Pharmacy*, first published in 1968. As my teaching commitments grew, so did my desire to use this as a source volume. However, I was surprised and disappointed to find that it was out of print.

Undoubtedly, there have been some classical texts on engineering principles applied to unit operation, most notably McCabe, Smith, and Harriott (*Unit Operations of Chemical Engineering*, McGraw-Hill). However, the uncomplicated manner in which Ganderton's book dealt with engineering principles gave it broad appeal. In 1996, Dr. Ganderton was kind enough to collaborate with me to reduce the original volume to two chapters for inclusion in the *Encyclopedia of Pharmaceutical Technology*. This achieved my major objective of making this material available to a new generation of pharmaceutical scientists and technologists. However, by inclusion in an encyclopedia, some of its earlier convenience was lost.

Imagine my delight to be invited by Marcel Dekker, Inc., to coauthor a revised and expanded volume on the subject of pharmaceutical process engineering. My enthusiasm was increased by the knowledge that Dr. Ganderton would again join me in preparing the material. We have updated the previous text and are privileged to place this volume back in print—a privilege that, in my opinion, it should never have been denied.

Pharmaceutical manufacturing entails the combination of a number of unit processes. The major processes are described in this text. The efficiency, quality, and economy of manufacturing depend on an understanding of the individual operations involved in processing. In many cases—unlike in other types of industrial processing—safety and efficacy of a therapeutic agent may be affected. This text constitutes a guide or introduction to the practical aspects of unit operations in pharmacy.

It is my sincere desire that this text should again find a role as a reference and review book for those new to the field of pharmaceutical manufacturing, from various scientific and engineering disciplines.

*Anthony J. Hickey*

Forty years ago it became clear that the contribution that a pharmaceutical scientist made to the manufacture of medicines would be enhanced by recruiting the principles used by chemical engineers. However, simple adoption was unsatisfactory because, in general, their texts were too complex and inadequately focused. For example, the study of mixing and dose uniformity, drying and product stability, and many others needed special consideration. For such reasons, *Unit Processes in Pharmacy* was written and published in the late 1960s. It enjoyed many years of success before it went out of print.

A generation later, Tony Hickey, who closely shares my enthusiasm for better understanding of pharmaceutical manufacture, suggested that the text should be brought up to date. This was a most flattering proposal and, recognizing the energy he has brought to the revision, I feel most privileged to see a new text with exactly the same ambitions as those that inspired me so many years ago.

*David Ganderton*

# Acknowledgments

This text would not have been possible without the contributions of Mr. Vasu Sethuraman. His endeavors with respect to the integration of chapters, production of figures, and copyediting are greatly appreciated. There is no doubt that his activities have contributed to the clarity and continuity of the book in its final form. I am grateful to Dr. Paul Pluta for sharing his thoughts on solid dosage forms and allowing me to use them in the relevant sections of the book.

The majority of the text of this book is based on a portion of David Ganderton's *Unit Processes in Pharmacy*, a book published in 1968 by Heineman Medical Books, Ltd., and now out of print. It is appropriate to acknowledge the contributions to that original volume.

The original text was the commission of Dr. D. M. Moulden. We acknowledge the considerable help given by his ideas, plans, and drafts. In addition, we thank Mr. Lan Boyd and Dr. John Hersey, who read and evaluated the manuscripts.

# Units and Dimensions

The pharmaceutical scientist is probably familiar with the units of centimeter (length), gram (mass), and second (time) or conventional Système Internationale (SI) units of meters, kilograms, and seconds. The engineer, on the other hand, will sometimes express his equations and calculations in units that suit the quantities he or she is measuring. To reconcile in small part this disparity, a brief account of units and dimensions follows.

Mass [M], length [L], time [T], and temperature [°] are four of six fundamental dimensions, the units of which have been fixed arbitrarily and from which all other units can be derived. The fundamental units chosen for this book are the kilogram (kg), meter (m), second (s), and kelvins (K). In many cases, derived units are self-evident. Examples are area ($m^2$) and velocity (m/s). Others are derived from established physical laws. Thus, a unit of force can be obtained from the law that relates force, $F$, to mass, $m$, and acceleration, $a$:

$$F = kma$$

where $k$ is a constant. If we choose our unit of force to be unity when the mass and acceleration are each unity, the units are consistent. On this basis, the unit of force is the newton (N). This is the force that will accelerate a kilogram mass at 1 $m/s^2$.

Similarly, a consistent expression of pressure (i.e., force per unit area) is newtons per square meter ($N/m^2$ or pascal, Pa). The expression exemplifies the use of multiples or fractions of the fundamental units to give derived units of practical value. A second example is dynamic viscosity $[M\ L^{-1}\ T^{-1}]$ when the consistent unit $kg \cdot m^{-1} \cdot s^{-1}$, which is enormous, is replaced by $kg \cdot m^{-1} \cdot hr^{-1}$, or even by the poise. Basic calculations using these quantities must then include conversion factors.

The relationship between weight and mass causes much confusion. A body falling freely due to its weight accelerates at $kg \cdot m/s^2$ ($g$ varies with height and latitude). Substituting 1 in the preceding equation gives $W = mg$, where $W$ is the weight of the body (in newtons). The weight of a body has the dimensions of force, and the mass of the body is given by

$$\text{Mass (kg)} = \frac{\text{weight (N)}}{\text{g(m/s}^2)}$$

The weight of a body varies with location; the mass does not. Problems arise when, as in many texts, the kilogram is used as a unit of mass and the weight of a kilogram as the unit of force. For example, an equation describing pressure drop in a pipe is

$$\Delta P = \frac{32ul\eta}{d^2}$$

when written in consistent units—$\Delta P$ as $N/m^2$, $\eta$ as $kg/m \cdot s$, $u$ as m/s, $l$ as m, and $d$ as m. If, however, the kilogram force was used (i.e., pressure was measured in $kg/m^2$), the equation must be

$$\Delta P = \frac{32ul\eta}{gd^2}$$

where $g = 9.8\ m/s^2$. In texts using this convention, the conversion factor $g$ appears in many equations.

The units of mass, length, and time commonly used in engineering heat transfer are the kilogram, the meter, and the second, respectively. Temperature, which forms a fourth fundamental unit, is measured in kelvins (K). The unit of heat is the joule (J), which is the quantity of heat required to raise the temperature of 1 g of water by 1 K. The rate of heat flow, $Q$, often referred to as the total heat flux, is therefore measured in J/s. The units of thermal conductivity are $J/m^2 \cdot s \cdot K/m$. This may also be written as $J/m \cdot s \cdot K$, although this form is less expressive of the meaning of the thermal conductivity.

# Contents

# 1

# Fluid Flow

## 1.1 SOME PROPERTIES OF FLUIDS

Fluids (liquids and gases) are a form of matter that cannot achieve equilibrium under an applied shear stress but deform continuously, or flow, as long as the shear stress is applied.

*Viscosity.* Viscosity is a property that characterizes the flow behavior of a fluid, reflecting the resistance to the development of velocity gradients within the fluid. Its quantitative significance may be explained by reference to Figure 1.1 A fluid is contained between two parallel planes each of area $A$ $m^2$ and distance $h$ m apart. The upper plane is subjected to a shear force of $F$ N and acquires a velocity of $u$ m $sec^{-1}$ relative to the lower plane. The shear stress, $t$, is $F/A$ N $m^{-2}$. The velocity gradient or rate of shear is given by $u/h$ or, more generally, by the differential coefficient $du/dy$, where $y$ is a distance measured in a direction perpendicular to the direction of shear. Since this term is described by the units velocity divided by a length, it has the dimension $T^{-1}$ or, in this example, reciprocal seconds. For gases, simple liquids, true solutions, and dilute disperse systems, the rate of shear is proportional to the shear stress. These systems are called Newtonian, and we can write

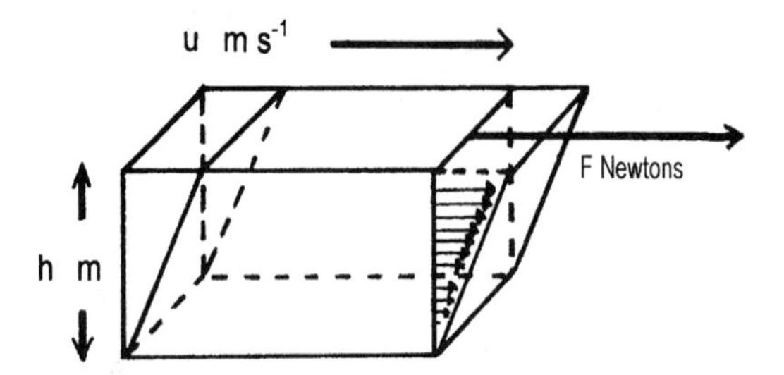


**FIGURE 1.1** Schematic of fluid flow depicting the applied force, velocity in the direction of motion, and thickness of fluid.

$$\frac{F}{A} = t = \eta \frac{du}{dy} \tag{1.1}$$

The proportionality constant η is the dynamic viscosity of the fluid: the higher its value, the lower the rates of shear induced by a given stress. The dimensions of dynamic viscosity are $M\ L^{-1}\ T^{-1}$. For the SI system of units, viscosity is expressed in $N \cdot s\ m^{-2}$. For the centimeter-gram-second (CGS) system, the unit of viscosity is the poise (P). One $N \cdot s\ m^{-2}$ is equivalent to 10 P. The viscosity of water at room temperature is about 0.01 P or 1 centipoise (cP). Pure glycerin at this temperature has a value of about 14 P. Air has a viscosity of $180 \times 10^{-6}$ P.

Complex disperse systems fail to show the proportionality described by equation 1.1, the viscosity increasing or, more commonly, decreasing with increase in the rate of shear. Viscosity may also depend upon the duration of shear and even on the previous treatment of the fluids. Such fluids are termed non-Newtonian.

Equation 1.1 indicates that wherever a velocity gradient is induced within a fluid, a shear stress will result. When the flow of a fluid parallel to some boundary is considered, it is assumed that no slip occurs between the boundary and the fluid, so the fluid molecules adjacent to the surface are at rest ($u = 0$). As shown in Figure 1.2, the velocity gradient $du/dy$ decreases from a maximum at the boundary ($y = 0$) to zero at some distance from the boundary ($y = y'$) when the velocity becomes equal to the undisturbed velocity of the fluid ($u = u'$). The shear stress must, therefore, increase from zero at this point to a maximum at the boundary. A shear stress, opposing the motion of the fluid and sometimes called fluid friction, is therefore developed at the boundary. The region limited by the dimension $y'$, in which flow of the fluid is perturbed by the boundary, is called the *boundary layer*. The structure of this layer greatly influences the rate at which heat is transferred from the

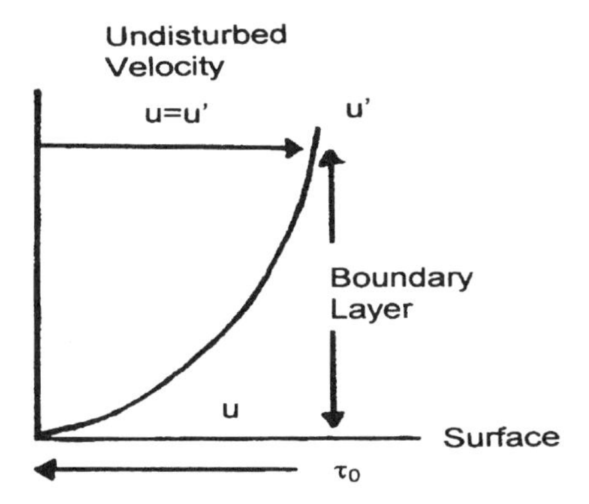


**FIGURE 1.2** Distribution of velocities at a boundary.

boundary to the fluid under the influence of a temperature gradient or the rate at which molecules diffuse from the boundary into the fluid under a concentration gradient. These topics are discussed in Chapters 2 and 3.

*Compressibility.* Deformation is not only a shear-induced phenomenon. If the stress is applied normally and uniformly over all boundaries, then fluids, like solids, decrease in volume. This decrease in volume yields a proportionate increase in density. Liquids can be regarded as incompressible, and changes of density with pressure can be ignored, with consequent simplification of any analysis. This is not possible in the study of gases if significant changes in pressure occur.

*Surface Tension.* Surface tension, a property confined to a free surface and, therefore, not applicable to gases, is derived from unbalanced intermolecular forces near the surface of a liquid. This may be expressed as the work necessary to increase the surface by unit area. Although not normally important, it can become so if the free surface is present in a passage of small-diameter orifice of tube. Capillary forces, determined by the surface tension and the curvature of the surface, may then be comparable in magnitude to other forces acting in the fluid. An example is found in the movement of liquid through the interstices of a bed of porous solids during drying.

## 1.2 FLUIDS AT REST—HYDROSTATICS

The study of fluids at rest is based on two principles:

1. Pressure intensity at a point, expressed as force per unit area, is the same in all directions.

2. Pressure is the same at all points in a given horizontal line in a continuous fluid.

The pressure, $P$, varies with depth, $z$, in a manner expressed by the hydrostatic equation:

$$dP = -\rho g\, dz \tag{1.2}$$

where $\rho$ is the density of the fluid and $g$ is the gravitational constant. Since water and most other liquids can be regarded as incompressible, the density is independent of the pressure, and integration between the limits $P_1$ and $P_2$, $z_1$ and $z_2$, gives

$$P_1 - P_2 = -\rho g(z_1 - z_2) \tag{1.3}$$

## 1.3 THE MEASUREMENT OF PRESSURE INTENSITY

Application of equation 1.3 to the column of liquid shown in Figure 1.3(a) gives

$$P_A - P_1 = -\rho gh$$

and (1.4)

$$P_1 = P_A + \rho gh$$

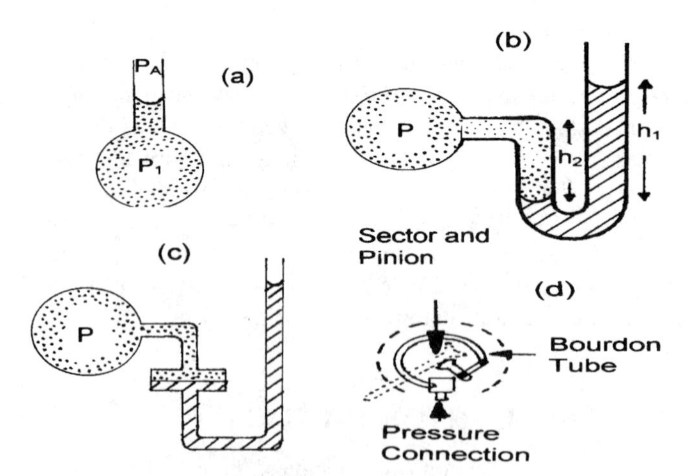


**FIGURE 1.3** Pressure measurement apparatus.

The density term should be the difference between the density of the liquid in the column and the density of the surrounding air. The latter is relatively small and this discrepancy can be ignored. $P_1$ is the absolute pressure at the point indicated, and $P_A$ is the atmospheric pressure. It is often convenient to refer to the pressure measured relative to atmospheric pressure, i.e., $P_1 - P_A$. This is called the gauge pressure and is equal to $\rho gh$. Pressure measured in SI units has units of N $m^{-2}$. Alternatively, the gauge pressure can be expressed as the height or head of a static liquid that would produce this pressure.

Figure 1.3(a) represents the simplest form of manometer, a device widely used for the measurement of pressure. It consists of a vertical tube tapped into the container of the fluid under study. In this form, it is confined to the pressure measurement of liquids. This device is unsuitable for the measurement of very large heads, due to unwieldy construction, or very small heads, due to low accuracy. The U-tube manometer, shown in Figure 1.3(b), may be used for the measurement of higher pressures with both liquids and gases. The density of the immiscible liquid in the U-tube, $\rho_1$ is greater than the density of the fluid in the container, $\rho_2$. The gauge pressure is given by

$$P = h_1\rho_1 g - h_2\rho_2 g$$

The disadvantage of reading two levels may be overcome by the modification in Figure 1.3(c). The cross-sectional area of one limb is many times larger than that of the other, and the vertical movement of the heavier liquid in the wider arm can be neglected and its level is assumed to be constant.

Sloping the reading arm of the manometer can increase the accuracy of the pressure determination, for small heads, with any of the manometers just described. The head is now derived from the distance moved along the tube and the angle of slope.

The Bourdon gauge, a compact instrument widely used for the measurement of pressure, differs in principle from the manometer. The fluid is admitted to a sealed tube of oval cross section, the shape of which is shown in Figure 1.3(d). The straightening of the tube under internal pressure is opposed by its elasticity. The movement to an equilibrium position actuates a recording mechanism. The gauge is calibrated by an absolute method of pressure measurement.

The principles of pressure measurement also apply to fluids in motion. However, the presence of the meter should minimize perturbation in flow. A calming section, in which a flow regime becomes stable, is present upstream from the pressure tapping, and the edge of the latter should be flush with the inside of the container to prevent flow disturbance.

## 1.4 FLUIDS IN MOTION

Streamlines are hypothetical entities without width that are drawn parallel at all points to the motion of the fluid. Figure 1.4 illustrates their use in depicting the flow of a fluid past a cylinder. If the flow at any position does not vary with time, it is steady and the streamlines retain their shape. In steady flow, a change in the spacing of the streamlines indicates a change in velocity because, by definition, no fluid can cross a streamline. In the regions on the upstream side of the cylinder, the velocity of the fluid is increasing. On the downstream side, the reverse occurs. The maximum velocity occurs in the fluid adjacent to regions B and D. At points A and C, the fluid is at rest. As the velocity increases, the pressure decreases. The pressure field around the cylinder is therefore the reverse of the velocity field. This statement may appear to contradict common experience. However, it follows from the principle of conservation of energy and finds expression in Bernoulli's theorem.

## 1.5 BERNOULLI'S THEOREM

At any point in flowing fluid, the total mechanical energy can be expressed in terms of the following components: potential energy, pressure energy, and kinetic energy. The potential energy of a body is its capacity to do work by reason of its position relative to some center of attraction. For a unit mass of fluid at a height $z$ above some reference level,

$$\text{Potential energy} = zg$$

where $g$ is the acceleration due to gravity.

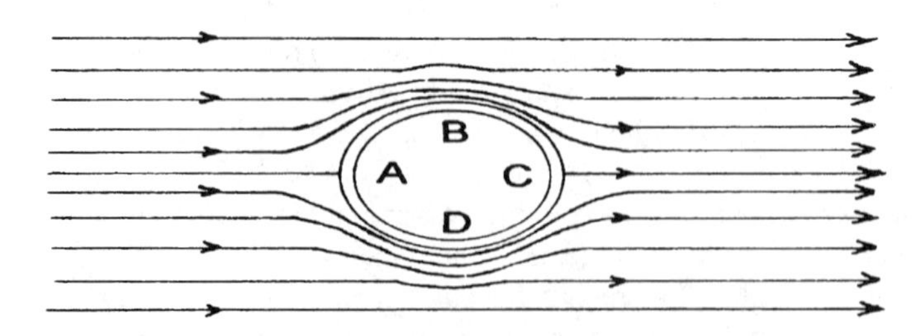


**FIGURE 1.4** Flow of a fluid past a cylinder.

The pressure energy or flow energy is an energy form peculiar to the flow of fluids. Figure 1.5 describes the flow of a volume of fluid, abdc, across the section $XX^1$. The work done and the energy acquired in transferring the fluid are the product of the pressure, $P$, and the volume. The volume of unit mass of the fluid is the reciprocal of the density, $\rho$. For an incompressible fluid, the density is not dependent on the pressure, so that for a unit mass of fluid:

$$\text{Pressure energy} = \frac{P}{\rho}$$

The kinetic energy is a form of energy possessed by a body by reason of its movement. If the mass of the body is $m$ and its velocity is $u$, the kinetic energy is $1/2\ mu^2$, and for a unit mass of fluid,

$$\text{Kinetic energy} = \frac{u^2}{2}$$

The total mechanical energy of a unit mass of fluid is, therefore,

$$\frac{u^2}{2} + \frac{P}{\rho} + zg$$

The mechanical energy at two points, A and B, will be the same if no energy is lost or gained by the system. Therefore, we can write

$$\frac{u_A^2}{2} + \frac{P_A}{\rho} + z_A g = \frac{u_B^2}{2} + \frac{P_B}{\rho} + z_B g \tag{1.5}$$

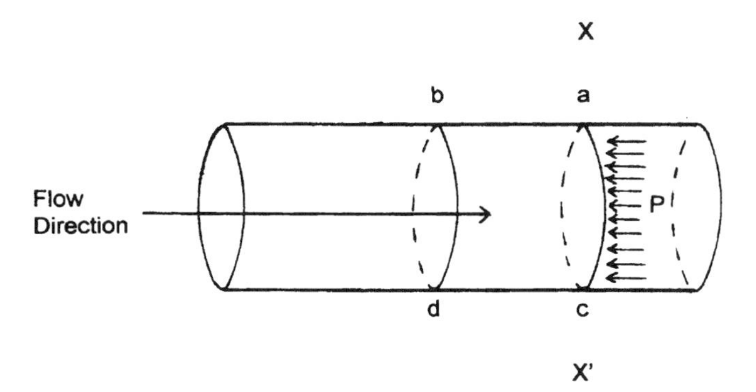


**FIGURE 1.5** Pressure energy of a fluid.

This relationship neglects the frictional degradation of mechanical energy that occurs in real systems. A fraction of the total energy is dissipated in overcoming the shear stresses induced by velocity gradients in the fluid. If the energy lost during flow between A and B is $E$, then equation 1.5 becomes

$$\frac{u_A^2}{2} + \frac{P_A}{\rho} + z_A g = \frac{u_B^2}{2} + \frac{P_B}{\rho} + z_B g + E \tag{1.6}$$

This is a form of Bernoulli's theorem, restricted in application to the flow of incompressible fluids. Each term is expressed in absolute units, such as N m $kg^{-1}$. The dimensions are $L^2\,T^{-2}$. In practice, each term is divided by $g(L\,T^{-2})$ to give the dimension of length. The terms are then referred to as velocity head, pressure head, potential head, and friction head, the sum giving the total head of the fluid:

$$\frac{u_A^2}{2g} + \frac{P_A}{\rho g} + z_A = \frac{u_B^2}{2g} + \frac{P_B}{\rho g} + z_B + \frac{E}{g} \tag{1.7}$$

The evaluation of the kinetic energy term requires consideration of the variation in velocity found in a direction normal to flow. The mean velocity, calculated by dividing the volumetric flow rate by the cross-sectional area of the pipe, lies between 0.5 and 0.82 times the maximum velocity found at the pipe axis. The value depends on whether flow is laminar or turbulent, terms which are described later. The mean kinetic energy, given by $u_{mean}^2/2$, differs from the true kinetic energy found by summation across the flow direction. The former can be retained, however, if a correction factor, $a$, is introduced. Then

$$\text{Velocity head} = \frac{u_{mean}^2}{2ga}$$

where $a$ has a value of 0.5 in laminar flow and approaches unity when flow is fully turbulent.

A second modification may be made to equation 1.5 if mechanical energy is added to the system at some point by means of a pump. If the work done, in absolute units, on a unit mass of fluid is $W$, then

$$\frac{W}{g} + \frac{u_A^2}{2g} + \frac{P_A}{\rho g} + z_A = \frac{u_B^2}{2g} + \frac{P_B}{\rho g} + z_B + \frac{E}{g}$$

or (1.8)

$$\frac{W}{g} + \frac{u_B^2 - u_A^2}{2g} + \frac{P_A}{\rho g} + z_A = \frac{u_B^2}{2g} + \frac{P_B}{\rho g} + z_B + \frac{E}{g}$$

The power required through a system at a certain rate may be calculated using equation 1.8 to drive a liquid. The changes in velocity, pressure, height, and the mechanical losses due to friction are each expressed as a head of liquid. The sum of heads, $\Delta H$, is the total head against which the pump must work. Therefore,

$$\frac{W}{g} = \Delta H$$

If the work performed and energy acquired by unit mass of fluid is $\Delta Hg$, then the power required to transfer mass $m$ in time $t$ is

$$\text{Power} = \frac{\Delta Hgm}{t}$$

Since the volume flowing in unit time, $Q$, is $m/\rho t$, then

$$\text{Power} = Q\Delta Hg\rho \tag{1.9}$$

## 1.6 FLOW MEASUREMENT

The Bernoulli theorem can also be applied to the measurement of flow rate. Consider the passage of an incompressible fluid through the constriction shown in Figure 1.6. The increase in kinetic energy as the velocity increases from $u_1$ to $u_2$ is derived from the pressure energy of the fluid, the pressure of which drops from $P_1$ to $P_2$, the latter being recorded by manometers. There is no change in height, and equation 1.5 can be rearranged to give

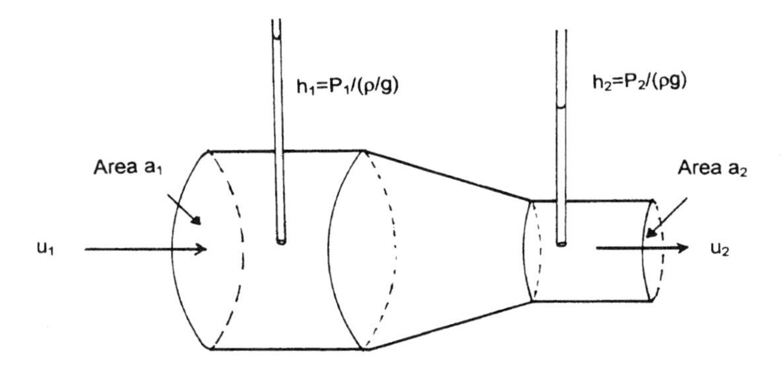


**FIGURE 1.6** Flow through a constriction.

$$\frac{u_2^2}{2} - \frac{u_1^2}{2} = \frac{P_1 - P_2}{\rho} \tag{1.10}$$

The volumetric flow rate $Q = u_1 a_1 = u_2 a_2$. Therefore, by rearrangement,

$$u_1 = u_2 \frac{a_2}{a_1}$$

Substituting for $u_1$ gives

$$\frac{u_2^2}{2} - \frac{u_2^2(a_2/a_1)}{2} = \frac{P_1 - P_2}{\rho}$$

and

$$\frac{u_2^2}{2}\left(1 - \frac{a_2^2}{a_1^2}\right) = \frac{P_1 - P_2}{\rho}$$

Therefore,

$$u_2 = \sqrt{\frac{2(P_1 - P_2)}{\rho(1 - a_2^2/a_1^2)}}$$

and

$$Q = a_2 \sqrt{\frac{2(P_1 - P_2)}{\rho(1 - a_2^2/a_1^2)}}$$

The derivation neglects the correction of kinetic energy due to nonuniformity of flow in both cross sections and the frictional degradation of energy during passage through the constriction. This is corrected by the introduction of a numerical coefficient, $C_D$, known as the coefficient of discharge. Therefore,

$$Q = C_D a_2 \sqrt{\frac{2(P_1 - P_2)}{\rho(1 - a_2^2/a_1^2)}} \tag{1.11}$$

The value of $C_D$ depends upon conditions of flow and the shape of the constriction. For a well-shaped constriction, such as that shown in Figure 1.6, it would vary between 0.95 and 0.99 for turbulent flow. The value is much lower in laminar flow because the kinetic energy correction is larger. The return of the fluid to the original velocity by means of a diverging section forms a flow-measuring device known as the Venturi meter.

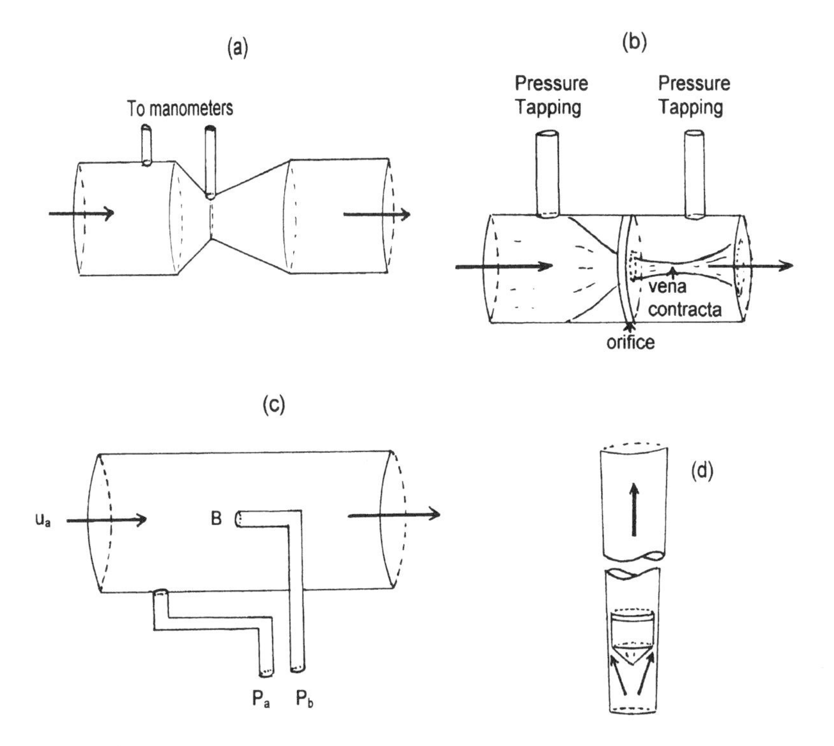


**FIGURE 1.7** Flow meters.

The *Venturi meter* is shown in Figure 1.7(a). The converging cone leads to the narrowest cross section, known as the throat. The change in pressure is measured across this part of the meter, and the volumetric flow rate found by substitution into equation 1.11. Values of the coefficient of discharge are given in the preceding paragraph. The diverging section, or diffuser, is designed to induce a gradual return to the original velocity. This minimizes eddy formation in the diffuser and permits the recovery of a large proportion of the increased kinetic energy as pressure energy. The permanent loss of head due to friction in both converging and diverging sections is small. The meter is therefore efficient.

When the minimization of energy degradation is less important, the gradual, economical return to the original velocity may be abandoned, compensation for loss of efficiency being found in a device that is simpler, cheaper, and more adaptable than the Venturi meter. The *orifice meter*, to which this statement applies, consists simply of a plate with an orifice. A representation of flow through the meter is shown in Figure 1.7(b), indicating convergence of the fluid stream after passage through the orifice to give a cross section of minimum area called the *vena contracta*. The downstream pressure tapping is made at this cross section. The volumetric flow rate is given by equation 1.11, for which $a_2$ is the jet area at the *vena contracta*. The measurement of $a_2$ is inconvenient. It is therefore related to the area of the orifice, $a_0$, which can be accurately measured, by the coefficient of contraction, $C_c$, defined by the relation

$$C_c = \frac{a_2}{a_0}$$

The coefficient of contraction, frictional losses between the tapping points, and kinetic energy corrections are absorbed in the coefficient of discharge. The volumetric flow rate is then

$$Q = a_0 \sqrt{\frac{2(P_1 - P_2)}{\rho(1 - a_0^2/a_1^2)}} \tag{1.12}$$

The term $1 - a_0^2/ a_1^2$ approaches unity if the orifice is small compared to the pipe cross section. Since $P_2 - P_1 = \Delta h \rho g$, where $\Delta h$ is the difference in head developed by the orifice, equation 1.12 reduces to

$$Q = a_0 C_D \sqrt{2 \Delta h g} \tag{1.13}$$

The value of $C_D$ for the orifice meter is about 0.6, varying with construction, the ratio $a_0/a_1$, and flow conditions within the meter. Due to its complexity, it cannot be calculated. After passage through the orifice, flow disturbance during retardation causes the dissipation of most of the excess kinetic energy as heat. The permanent loss of head is therefore high, increasing as the ratio $a_0/a_1$ falls and ultimately reaching the differential head produced within the meter. When constructional requirements and methods of installation are followed, the correcting coefficients can be derived from charts. Alternatively, the meters can be calibrated.

The Bernoulli theorem may be used to determine the change in pressure caused by retardation of fluid at the upstream side of a body immersed in a fluid stream. This principle is applied in the use of the *Pitot tube*, shown in Figure 1.7(c). The fluid velocity is reduced from $u_a$, the velocity of the fluid filament in alignment with the tube, to zero at B, a position known as the stagnation point. The pressure, $P_b$, is measured at this point by the method shown in Figure 1.7(c). The undisturbed pressure, $P_a$, is measured in this example with a tapping point in the wall connected to a manometer. Since the velocity at B is zero, equation 1.10 reduces to

$$\frac{u_a^2}{2} = \frac{P_b - P_a}{\rho}$$

and $u_a$ can be calculated. Since only a local velocity is measured, variation of velocity in a section can be studied by altering the position of the tube. This procedure must be used if the flow rate in a pipe is to be measured. The mean velocity is derived from velocities measured at different distances from the wall. This derivation and the low-pressure differential developed render the Pitot tube less accurate than either the Venturi tube or the orifice meter for flow measurement. However, the tube is small in comparison with the pipe diameter and therefore produces no appreciable loss of head.

The *rotameter* (a variable-area meter), shown in Figure 1.7(d), is commonly used, giving a direct reading of flow rate by the position of a small float in a vertical, calibrated glass tube through which the fluid is flowing. The tube is internally tapered toward the lower end so that the annulus between float and wall varies with the position of the float. Acceleration of the fluid through the annulus produces a pressure differential across the position of the float and an upward force upon it. At the equilibrium position, which may be stabilized by a slow rotation of the float, the weight force acting on the float balances this upward force. If increasing the rate of flow disturbs equilibrium, the balance of weight force and pressure differential is produced by movement of the float upward to a position at which the area of the annulus is bigger. For accurate measurement, the rotameter is calibrated with the fluid to be metered. Its use is then restricted to that fluid. A theoretical derivation of flow rate is also available.

## 1.7 LAMINAR AND TURBULENT FLOWS

The translation of the energy of flow from one form to another has been described with little reference to the actual nature of flow. Flow of fluids can be laminar (and may be depicted by streamlines) or turbulent, terms that are best introduced by describing a series of simple experiments performed in 1883 by Osborne Reynolds. The apparatus, shown in Figure 1.8, consisted of a straight glass tube through which the fluid was allowed to flow. The nature of flow was examined by introducing a dye into the axis of the tube. At low speeds, the dye formed a coherent thread that grew very little in thickness

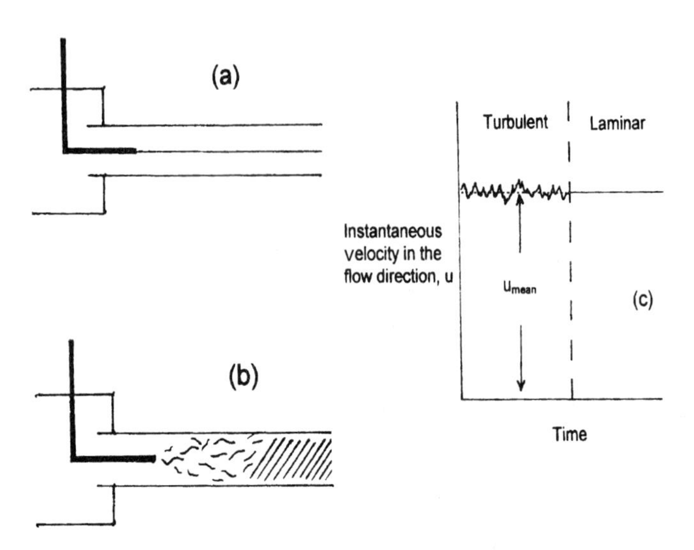


**FIGURE 1.8** The Reynolds experiment (diagrammatic).

with distance down the tube. However, with progressive increase in speed, the line of dye first began to waver and then to break up. Secondary motions, crossing and recrossing the general flow direction, were clearly revealed. Finally, at very high speeds, no filament of dye could be detected, and mixing to a dilute color was almost instantaneous. In this experiment, flow changed from laminar to turbulent, the change occurring at a critical speed. In the former, flow was ordered, always moving parallel to the walls of the tube. Generalizing, in laminar flow the instantaneous velocity at a point is always the same as the mean velocity in both magnitude and direction. In turbulent flow, order is lost and irregular motions are imposed upon the main steady motion of the fluid. At any instant of time, the fluid velocity at a point varies in magnitude and direction, having components perpendicular, as well as parallel, to the direction of net flow. Over time, these fluctuations even out to give the net velocity in the direction of flow.

In turbulent flow, rapidly fluctuating velocities produce high-velocity gradients within the fluid. Proportionately large shear stresses are developed, and to overcome them mechanical energy is degraded and dissipated in the form of heat. The degradation of energy in laminar flow is much smaller.

The random motions of turbulent flow provide a mechanism of momentum transfer not present in laminar flow. If a variation in velocity occurs across a fluid stream, as in a pipe, a quantity of fast-moving fluid can move across the flow direction to a slower-moving region, increasing the momentum of the latter. A corresponding movement must take place in the reverse direction elsewhere, and a complementary set of rotational movements, called an eddy, is imposed on the main flow. This is a powerful mechanism for equalizing momentum. By the same mechanism, any variation in the concentration of a component is quickly eliminated. Admitting dye to the fluid stream in Reynolds' original experiment showed this. Similarly, the gross mixing of turbulent flow quickly erases variations in temperature.

The turbulent mechanism that carries motion, heat, or matter from one part of the fluid to another is absent in laminar flow. The shear stress arises from the variations in velocity; i.e., the viscosity brings about momentum transfer. Similarly, heat and matter can only be transferred across streamlines on a molecular scale, heat by conduction and matter by diffusion. These mechanisms, which are present but less important in turbulent flow, are comparatively slow. Velocity, temperature, and concentration gradients are, therefore, much greater than in turbulent flow.

## 1.8 LIQUIDS FLOW IN PIPES

The many pharmaceutical processes that involve the transfer of a liquid from one place to another confer great importance on the study of flow in pipes. This study permits the evaluation of pressure loss due to friction in a simple pipe and assesses the additional effects of pipe roughness, changes in diameter, bends, exits, and entrances. When the total pressure drop due to friction is known for the system, the equivalent head can be derived and the power requirement for driving a liquid through the system can be calculated from equation 1.9.

### 1.8.1 Streamline Flow in a Tube

The mathematical analysis of streamline flow in a simple tube is complete and results in the expression known as Poiseuille's law, one form of which is

$$Q = \frac{\pi \Delta P d^4}{128 \eta l} \tag{1.14}$$

where $Q$ is the volumetric flow rate or discharge, $\Delta P$ is the pressure drop

$$\int_{0}^{u} du = -\frac{\Delta \Pr}{2\eta l} \int_{R}^{r} r dr$$

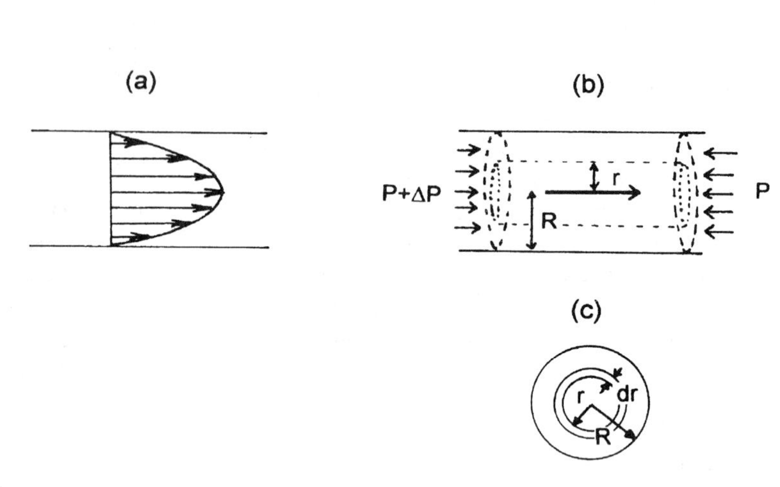


**FIGURE 1.9** Streamline flow: velocity distribution in a pipe.

across the tube, $d$ and $l$ are the diameter and length of the tube, respectively, and $\eta$ is the fluid viscosity.

Whether flow in the tube is streamline or turbulent, an infinitesimally thin stationary layer is found at the wall. The velocity increases from zero at this point to a maximum at the axis of the tube. For streamline flow, the velocity profile is presented in Figure 1.9(a). The velocity gradient, $du/dr$, varies from a maximum at the wall to zero at the axis. In flow through a tube, the rate of shear is equal to the velocity gradient, so that equation 1.1 dictates the same variation of shear stress.

To derive Poiseuille's law, the form of the velocity profile must first be established. Consider the fluid contained within a radius $r$ flowing in a tube of radius $R$. This is shown in Figure 1.9(b). If the pressure drop across length $l$ is $\Delta P$, the force attributed to the applied pressure driving this section is $\Delta P \pi r^2$. If flow is steady, this force can only be balanced by opposing viscous forces acting on the ''wall'' of the section. This force, the product of the shear stress $\pi$ and the area over which it acts, is $2t\pi l$. The expression given by equating these forces is

$$t = \frac{\Delta P r^2}{2l}$$

Substituting from equation 1.1 gives

$$-\frac{du}{dr} = \frac{\Delta Pr}{2\eta l}$$

The velocity gradient is negative because $u$ decreases as $r$ increases. When $r = R$, $u = 0$. Integrating gives

$$\int_0^u du = -\frac{\Delta Pr}{2\eta l}\int_R^r r\,dr$$

Therefore,

$$u = \frac{\Delta P}{2\eta l}\left(\frac{R^2 - r^2}{2}\right) \tag{1.15}$$

This relation shows that the velocity distribution across the tube is parabolic. For such a distribution, the maximum velocity is twice the mean velocity. The volumetric flow rate across the annular section between $r$ and $r + dr$, shown in Figure 1.9(c), is

$$Q = 2\pi r \cdot dr \cdot u$$

Substituting for $u$ from equation 1.15 gives

$$Q = \frac{\Delta P\pi}{2\eta l}(R^2 r - r^3)\,dr$$

The total volumetric flow rate is the integral between the limits $r = R$ and $r = 0$:

$$Q = \frac{\Delta P\pi}{2\eta l}\int_0^R (R^2 r - r^3)\,dr$$

$$= \frac{\Delta P\pi}{2\eta l}\left[\frac{R^2 r^2}{2} - \frac{r^4}{4}\right]_0^R$$

Therefore,

$$Q = \frac{\Delta P\pi R^4}{8\eta l} = \frac{\Delta P\pi d^4}{128\eta l} \tag{1.14}$$

where $d$ is the diameter of the tube. Since $Q = u_{mean}\pi d^2/4$, substitution and rearrangement give

$$\Delta P = \frac{32u_{mean}\eta l}{d^2} \tag{1.16}$$

### 1.8.2 Dimensional Analysis and Flow through a Tube: A General Approach

The utility of equation 1.16 for evaluating the loss of pressure due to friction in a tube is limited because streamline conditions are rare in practice. The theoretical analysis of turbulent flow, however, is incomplete, and experiments with fluids are necessary for the development of satisfactory relations between the controlling variables. In such experiments, it is often not possible to study the relation of two variables, one in terms of the other, while other variables are temporarily held constant. Dimensional analysis is a procedure in which the interaction of variables is presented in such a way that the effect of each variable can be assessed.

The method is based on the requirement that the dimensions of all terms of a physically meaningful equation are the same; i.e., an equation must be dimensionally homogeneous. This principle may be usefully illustrated by reference to equation 1.14 written in the form

$$Q \alpha \frac{\Delta P d''}{\eta l}$$

Rewriting in basic units of mass, length, and time, and using the symbol [ ] to represent dimensions of, $[Q] = [\mathrm{L}^3\,\mathrm{T}^{-1}]$, $[\Delta P] = [\mathrm{M\,L}^{-1}\,\mathrm{T}^{-2}]$, $[d^n] = [\mathrm{L}^n]$, and $[\eta] = [\mathrm{M\,L}^{-1}\,\mathrm{T}^{-1}]$. Equating gives

$$[\mathrm{L}^3\,\mathrm{T}^{-2}] = \left[\frac{\mathrm{M\,L}^{-1}\,\mathrm{T}^{-2}\cdot\mathrm{L}^n}{\mathrm{M\,L}^{-1}\,\mathrm{T}^{-1}\cdot\mathrm{L}}\right] = [\mathrm{L}^{n-1}\,\mathrm{T}^{-1}]$$

[M] and [T] are correct, as they must be. Equating for [L] gives $[\mathrm{L}^3] = [\mathrm{L}^{n-1}]$, from which $n = 4$.

If no previous knowledge of the combined form of the variables that determine $Q$ is available, dimensional analysis can be applied in the following way. The dependence of $Q$ on $\Delta P$, $l$, $d$, and $\eta$ can be written as

$$Q = f(\Delta P, l, d, \eta)$$

The function $f$ can be expressed as a series, each term of which is the product of the independent variables raised to suitable powers. Taking the first term of the series gives

$$Q = N \cdot \Delta P^{w} \cdot l^{x} \cdot d^{y} \cdot \eta^{z}$$

where $N$ is a numerical factor (dimensionless). Rewriting terms as $[Q] = [\mathrm{L}^3\ \mathrm{T}^{-1}]$, $[\Delta P^w] = [\mathrm{M}^w\ \mathrm{L}^{-w}\ \mathrm{T}^{-2w}]$, $[l^x] = [\mathrm{L}^x]$, $[d^y] = [\mathrm{L}^y]$, and $[\eta^z] = [\mathrm{M}^z\ \mathrm{L}^{-z}\ \mathrm{T}^{-z}]$, the equation $[Q] = [\Delta P^w \cdot l^x \cdot d^y \cdot \eta^z]$ becomes $[\mathrm{L}^3\ \mathrm{T}^{-1}] = [\mathrm{M}^w\ \mathrm{L}^{-w}\ \mathrm{T}^{-2w} \cdot \mathrm{L}^x \cdot \mathrm{L}^y \cdot \mathrm{M}^z\ \mathrm{L}^{-z}\ \mathrm{T}^{-z}]$.

Equating powers of M, L, and $T$ gives the system

$$\begin{aligned} &\mathrm{M}: & 0 &= w + z \\ &\mathrm{L}: & 3 &= -w + x + y - z \\ &\mathrm{T}: & -1 &= -2w - z \end{aligned}$$

Since four unknowns are present in three simultaneous equations, three may be determined in terms of the fourth. Solving gives $w = 1$, $z = -1$, and $x + y = 3$. Expressing $y$ as $3 - x$; one gets

$$\begin{aligned} Q &= N\frac{\Delta P}{\eta} d^{3-x} l^{x} \\ &= N\frac{\Delta P d^3}{\eta}\left(\frac{l}{d}\right)^{x} \end{aligned} \tag{1.17}$$

The first part of the example demonstrates the use of dimensions as a partial check on the derivation or completeness of a solution. In the second part, a solution, although incomplete, gives considerable information about discharge of a fluid in streamline flow and its relation to pressure drop, viscosity, and the geometry of the pipe without any theoretical or experimental analysis. For example, if two tubes had the same ratio $l/d$, the values of $Q\eta/d^3\Delta P$ would also be the same.

Since the exponent $x$ in equation 1.17 is indeterminate, the term in brackets must be dimensionless. Unlike the lengths from which it is derived, it is a pure number and needs no system of units for meaningful expression. Its value is, therefore, independent of the units chosen for its measurement, providing, of course, that the systems of measurement are not mixed. The equation may therefore be presented as the relation between two dimensionless groups:

$$\frac{Q\eta}{d^3 \Delta P} = N\left(\frac{l}{d}\right)^{x}$$

or, since a series of power terms will, in general, form the original unknown function, each of which has different values of $N$ and $x$,

$$\frac{Q\eta}{d^3 \Delta P} = f\left(\frac{l}{d}\right) \tag{1.18}$$

The study of frictional losses at the wall of a pipe is facilitated by dimensional analysis. The shear stress—that is, the force opposing motion of the fluid acting on each unit of area of the pipe, $R$—is determined, for a given pipe surface, by the velocity of the fluid, $u$, the diameter of the pipe, $d$, the viscosity of the fluid, $\eta$, and the fluid density, $\rho$. The equation of dimensions is

$$[R] = [u^0 \cdot d^q \cdot \eta^r \cdot \rho^s]$$

Therefore,

$$\mathrm{M\,L^{-1}\,T^{-2} = L^{p}\,T^{-p} \cdot L^{q} \cdot M^{r}\,L^{-r}\,T^{-r} \cdot M^{s}\,L^{-3s}}$$

Equating M, L, and T, one gets

$$\text{M:} \quad 1 = r + s$$

$$\text{L:} \quad -1 = p + q - r - 3s$$

$$\text{T:} \quad -2 = -p - r$$

Solving for $p$, $r$, and $s$ in terms of $q$ gives $r = -q$, $s = 1 + q$, and $p = 2 + q$. Therefore,

$$R = N \cdot u^{2+q} \cdot d^q \cdot \eta^{-q} \cdot \rho^{1+q} = N\,\rho u^2 \left(\frac{ud\rho}{\eta}\right)$$

where $N$ is a numerical factor. Generalizing, $R/\rho u^2$, which is the friction factor, is a function of a dimensionless combination of $u$, $d$, $\eta$, and $\rho$. This combination gives a parameter known as the Reynolds number, Re. Therefore,

$$\frac{R}{\rho u^2} = f(\mathrm{Re}) \tag{1.19}$$

The form of this relation must largely be determined by experiment. If the friction factor, $R/\rho u^2$, is plotted against Re, all data lie on a single curve which, although restricted to a particular pipe surface, will apply to all fluids, all pipe diameters, and all velocities.

In turbulent flow, the shear stress at the wall depends upon the surface, the value being higher for a rough pipe than for a smooth pipe when flow conditions are otherwise the same. Equation 1.19 therefore yields a family of curves when pipes of differing surface condition are used. This is rationalized by the introduction of another dimensionless group, $e/d$, in which $e$ is a linear dimension expressing roughness. Values of $e$ are known for many materials.

The complete dimensionless correlation, plotted on logarithmic coordinates so that widely varying conditions are covered, is given in Figure 1.10. The curve can be divided into four regions. When Re $< 2000$, flow is streamline and the equation of the line in this region is $R/\rho u^2 = 8/\text{Re}$. This is simply another form of Poiseuille's law. The friction factor is independent of the roughness of the pipe and all data fall on a single line.

When Re lies between 2000 and 3000, flow normally becomes turbulent. The exact value of the transition depends upon the idiosyncrasies of the system. For example, in a smooth pipe, streamline conditions will persist at higher Reynolds number than in a pipe in which disturbances are created by surface roughness.

At higher values of Re, flow becomes increasingly turbulent to give a region in which the friction factor is a function of Re and surface roughness. Ultimately, this merges with a region in which the friction factor is indepen-

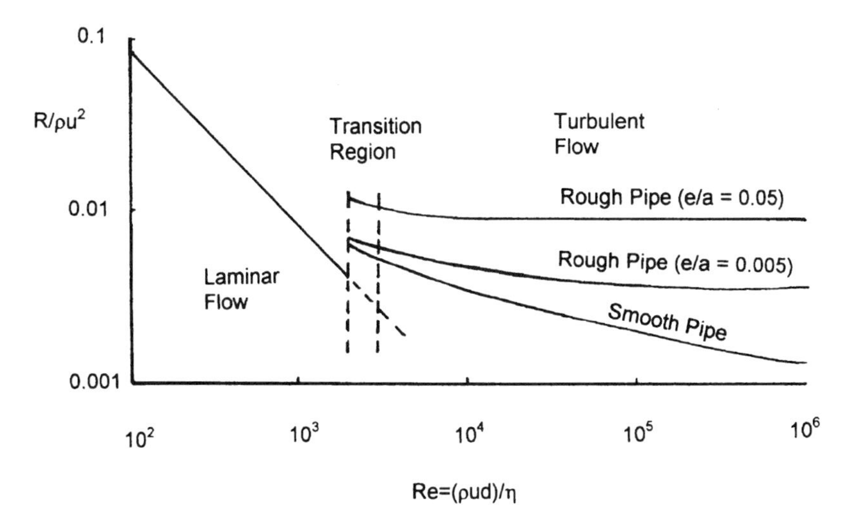


**FIGURE 1.10** Pipe friction chart.

dent of Re. Flow is fully turbulent and, for a given surface, the shear stress at the pipe wall is proportional to the square of the fluid velocity. The onset of the fourth region occurs at a lower Re in rough pipes.

The essential difference between laminar flow and turbulent flow has already been described. In a pipe, the enhanced momentum transfer of the latter modifies the velocity distribution. In laminar flow, this distribution is parabolic. In turbulent flow, a much greater equalization of velocity occurs, the velocity profile becomes flatter, and high-velocity gradients are confined to a region quite close to the wall. In both cases, the boundary layer, the region in which flow is perturbed by the presence of the boundary, extends to the pipe axis and completely fills the tube. In laminar conditions, the structure of the layer is quite simple, layers of fluid sliding one over another in an orderly fashion. In turbulent flow, however, division can be made into three regimes: (1) The core of fluid is turbulent. (2) In a thin layer at the wall a fraction of a millimeter thick, laminar conditions persist. This is called the laminar sublayer and it is separated from the turbulent core by (3) a buffer layer in which transition from turbulent flow to laminar flow occurs.

This description of the turbulent boundary layer applies generally to the flow of fluids over surfaces. The properties of this layer are central in many aspects of the flow of fluids. In addition, these properties determine the rate at which heat or mass is transferred to or from the boundary. These subjects are described in Chapters 2 and 3.

## 1.9 THE SIGNIFICANCE OF REYNOLDS' NUMBER, RE

In Reynolds' experiment, described previously, progressive increase in velocity caused a change from laminar flow to turbulent flow. This change would also have occurred if the diameter of the tube was increased while maintaining the velocity, or if the fluid was replaced by one of higher density. On the other hand, an increase in viscosity could promote a change in the opposite direction. Obviously, all these factors are simultaneously determining the nature of flow. These factors, which alone determine the character of flow, combine to give some value of Re. This indicates that the forces acting on some fluid element have a particular pattern. If some other geometrically similar system has the same Re, the fluid will be subject to the same force pattern.

More specifically, the Reynolds number describes the ratio of the inertia and viscous or frictional forces. The higher the Reynolds number, the greater will be the relative contribution of inertial effects. At very low Re, viscous

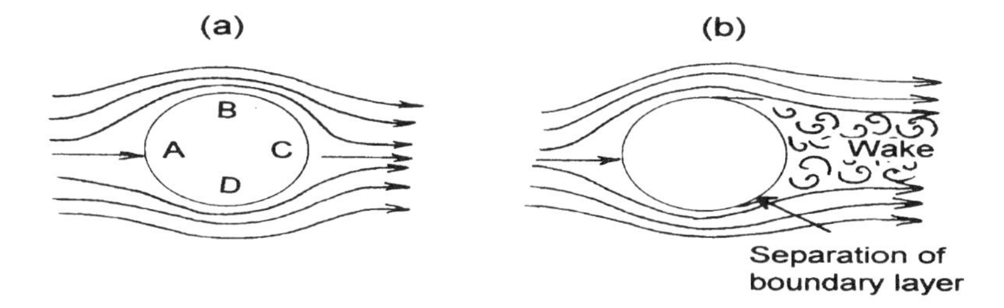


**FIGURE 1.11** Flow of a fluid past a cylinder.

effects predominate and the contribution of inertial forces can be ignored. A clear example of the changing contributions of viscous and inertia or momentum effects and the resulting changes in the flow pattern is given in Figure 1.11. A Reynolds number can also characterize flow in this quite different system.

## 1.10 CALCULATION OF THE PRESSURE DROP IN A PIPE DUE TO FRICTION

If the volumetric flow rate of a liquid of density $\rho$ and viscosity $\eta$ through a pipe of diameter $d$ is $Q$, the derivation of the mean velocity, $u$, from the flow rate and pipe area completes the data required for calculating Re. If the pipe roughness factor is known, the equivalent value of $R/\rho u^2$ can be determined from Figure 1.10, and the shear stress at the pipe wall can be calculated. The total frictional force opposing motion is the product of $R$ and the surface area of the pipe, $\pi dl$, where $l$ is the pipe length. If the unknown pressure drop across the pipe is $\Delta P$, the force driving the fluid through the pipe is $\Delta P$ $(\pi d^2/4)$. Equating pressure force and frictional force gives

$$\Delta P \frac{\pi d^2}{4} = R\pi dl$$

Therefore,

$$\Delta P = \frac{4Rl}{d} \tag{1.20}$$

Division by $\rho g$ gives the pressure loss as a friction head. This form is used in equations 1.7 and 1.8.

## 1.11 FLOW IN TUBES OF NONCIRCULAR CROSS SECTION

Discussion of flow in pipes has been restricted to pipes of circular cross section. The previous exposition may be applied to turbulent flow in noncircular ducts by introducing a dimension equivalent to the diameter of a circular pipe. This is known as the mean hydraulic diameter, $d_m$, which is defined as four times the cross-sectional area divided by the wetted perimeter. The following examples are given:

For a square channel of side $b$:

$$d_m = \frac{4b^2}{4b} = b$$

For an annulus of outer radius $r_1$ and inner radius $r_2$:

$$\frac{4(\pi r_1^2 - \pi r_2^2)}{2\pi r_1 + 2\pi r_2} = 2(r_1 - r_2)$$

This simple modification does not apply to laminar flow in noncircular ducts.

## 1.12 FRICTIONAL LOSSES AT PIPE FITTINGS

Losses occur at the various fittings and valves used in practical systems in addition to the friction losses at the wall of a straight pipe. In general, these losses are derived from sudden changes in the magnitude or direction of flow induced by changes in geometry. They can be classified as loss due to a sudden contraction or enlargement, losses at entrance or exit, and loss due to pipe curvature. Losses can be conveniently expressed as a length of straight pipe offering the same resistance. This is usually in the form of a number of pipe diameters. For example, the loss at a right-angled elbow is equivalent to a length of straight pipe equal to 40 diameters. The sum of the equivalent lengths of all fittings and valves is then added to the actual pipe length and the total frictional loss is estimated by equation 1.20.

## 1.13 MOTION OF BODIES IN A FLUID

When a body moves relative to a fluid in which it is immersed, resistance to motion is encountered and a force must be exerted in the direction of relative body movement. The opposing drag force is made up from two components:

viscous drag and form drag. This may be explained by reference to Figure 1.11, which describes the flow past a body, in this case a cylinder with axis normal to the page, by means of streamlines. As mentioned, streamlines are hypothetical lines drawn tangential at all points to the motion of the fluid. Flow past the cylinder immobilizes the fluid layer in contact with the surface, and the induced velocity gradients result in a shear stress or viscous drag on the surface. The crowding of streamlines on the upstream face of the cylinder to points B and D indicates an increase in velocity and, therefore, a decrease in pressure. If there is to be no inertial force acting on the cylinder, the flow pattern and momentum changes on the downstream surface must be exactly reversed. This is shown in Figure 1.11(a), and the entire force opposing relative motion of the cylinder and fluid is viscous drag. However, conditions of increasing pressure and decreasing velocity that exist on the downstream surface may cause the boundary layer to separate. The region between the breakaway streamlines—the wake—is occupied by eddies and vortices, and the flow pattern shown in Figure 1.11(b) is established. The kinetic energy of the accelerated fluid is dissipated and not recovered as pressure energy on the downstream surface. Under these conditions, there is a second component to the force opposing relative motion. This is known as form drag. Its contribution to the total drag increases as the velocity increases.

Once again, viscous and inertial forces are operating to determine the flow pattern and drag force on a body moving relative to a fluid. Reynolds number, which expresses their ratio, is used as a parameter to predict flow behavior. The relation between the drag force and its controlling variables is presented in a manner similar to that employed for flow in a pipe. If we consider a sphere moving relative to a fluid, the projected area normal to flow is where $d$ is the diameter of the sphere. The drag force acting on unit projected area, $R'$, is determined by the fluid's velocity, $u$, viscosity, $\eta$, and density, $\rho$, and by $d$. Dimensional analysis yields the relation

$$\frac{R'}{\rho u^2} = f(\mathrm{Re}') = f\left(\frac{ud\rho}{\eta}\right) \tag{1.21}$$

This form of Reynolds number, Re′, employs the sphere diameter as the linear dimension. With the exception of an analysis at very low Reynolds numbers, the form of this function is established by experiment. Results are presented on logarithmic coordinates in Figure 1.12. When $\mathrm{Re}' \lesssim 0.2$, viscous forces are solely responsible for drag on the sphere and equation 1.21 is

$$\frac{R'}{\rho u^2} = \frac{12}{\mathrm{Re}'}$$

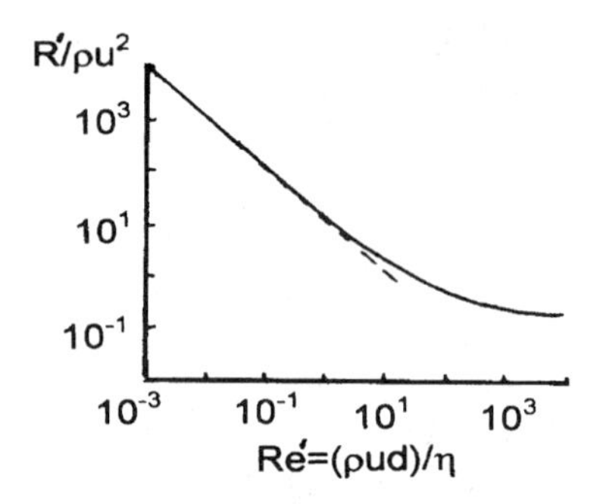


**FIGURE 1.12** $R'/\rho u^2$ vs. Re′ for a smooth sphere.

Therefore,

$$\begin{aligned}\text{Total drag force} &= R' \frac{\pi d^2}{4} \\ &= \rho u^2 \frac{12}{\text{Re}'}\left(\frac{\pi d^2}{4}\right) \qquad (1.22) \\ &= 3\pi\eta d u\end{aligned}$$

This is the normal form of Stokes' law.

At larger values of Re′, the experimental curve progressively diverges from this relation, ultimately becoming independent of Re′ and giving $R'/\rho u^2 \approx 0.22$. As Re′ increases, the form drag increases, ultimately becoming solely responsible for the force opposing motion.

For nonspherical particles the analysis employs the diameter of a sphere of equivalent volume. A correction factor, which depends upon the shape of the body and its orientation in the fluid, must then be applied.

An important application of this analysis is the estimation of the speed at which particles settle in a fluid. Under the action of gravity, the particle accelerates until the weight force, $mg$, is exactly balanced by the opposing drag. The body then falls at a constant terminal velocity $u$. Equating weight and drag forces gives

$$mg = \frac{\pi}{6} d^3 (\rho_s - \rho) g = R' \frac{\pi d^2}{4} \qquad (1.23)$$

where $\rho_s$ is the density of the particle.

For a sphere falling under streamline conditions ($\mathrm{Re}' < 0.2$), $R' = \rho u^2 (12/\mathrm{Re}')$. Substituting in equation 1.23, we obtain

$$u = \frac{d^2(\rho_s - \rho)g}{18\eta} \tag{1.24}$$

This expression follows more simply from the equation $mg = 3\,\pi\eta du$.

## 1.14 FLOW OF FLUIDS THROUGH PACKED BEDS

Fluids flow analysis through a permeable bed of solids is widely applied in filtration, leaching, and several other processes. A first approach may be made by assuming that the interstices of the bed correspond to a large number of discrete, parallel capillaries. If flow is streamline, the volumetric flow rate, $Q$, is given for a single capillary by equation 1.14:

$$Q = \frac{\Delta P \pi d^4}{128\eta l} \tag{1.14}$$

where $l$ is the capillary length, $d$ is capillary diameter, $\Delta P$ is the pressure drop across the capillary, and $\eta$ is the fluid viscosity. The capillary length will exceed the depth of the bed by an amount that depends upon its tortuosity. The bed depth $L$ is, however, proportional to $l$, so

$$Q = \frac{\Delta P d^4}{k\eta L}$$

where $k$ is a constant for a particular bed. If the area of the bed is $A$ and contains $n$ capillaries per unit area, the total flow rate is given by

$$Q = \frac{\Delta P d^4 n A}{k\eta L}$$

Although $n$ and $d$ are not normally known, they have certain values for a given bed so that

$$Q = KA\frac{\Delta P}{\eta L} \tag{1.25}$$

where $K = d^4 n/k$ is a permeability coefficient and $1/K$ is the specific resistance. Its value characterizes a particular bed.

The postulate of discrete capillaries precludes valid comment on the factors that determine the permeability coefficient. Channels are not discrete but are interconnected in a random manner. Nevertheless, the resistance to the passage of fluid must depend on the number and dimensions of the channels. These quantities can be expressed in terms of the fraction of the bed that is void—that is, the porosity—and the manner in which the void fraction is distributed. With reference to a specific example, water flows more easily through a bed with a porosity of 40% than through a bed of the same material with a porosity of 25%. It also flows more quickly through a bed of coarse particles than through a bed of fine particles packed to the void fraction or porosity. The latter effect can be expressed in terms of the surface area offered to the fluid by the bed. This property is inversely proportional to the size of the particles forming the bed. Permeability increases as the porosity increases and the total surface of the bed decreases, and these factors may be combined to give the hydraulic diameter, $d'$, of an equivalent channel, defined by

$$d' = \frac{\text{Volume of voids}}{\text{Total surface of material forming bed}}$$

The volume of voids is the porosity, and the volume of solids is $1 - \varepsilon$. If the specific surface area, that is, the surface area of unit volume of solids, is $S_0$, the total surface presented by unit volume of the bed is $S_0(1 - \varepsilon)$. Therefore;

$$d' = \frac{\varepsilon}{S_0(1 - \varepsilon)} \tag{1.26}$$

Under laminar flow conditions, the rate at which a fluid flows through this equivalent channel is given by Poiseuille's equation, 1.14:

$$Q = \frac{\Delta P d'^4}{k \eta L}$$

The velocity, $u'$, in the channel is derived by dividing the volumetric flow rate by the area of the channel, $k'' d'^2$. Combining the constants produces

$$u' = \frac{Q}{k'' d'^2} = \frac{\Delta P d'^4}{k'' \eta L}$$

This velocity, when averaged over the entire area of the bed, solids, and voids, gives the lower value $u$. These velocities are related by the equation $u = u'\varepsilon$. Therefore,

$$\frac{u}{\varepsilon} = \frac{\Delta P d'^2}{k'' \eta L}$$

Substituting for $d'$ by means of equation 1.26 gives

$$\frac{u}{\varepsilon} = \frac{\Delta P}{k''\eta L} \frac{\varepsilon^2}{(1 - \varepsilon)^2 S_0^2}$$

and

$$u = \frac{\Delta P}{k''\eta L} \frac{\varepsilon^3}{(1 - \varepsilon)^2 S_0^2} \tag{1.27}$$

In this equation, known after its originator as Kozeny's equation, the constant $k''$ has a value of $5 \pm 0.5$. Since $Q = uA$, where $A$ is the area of the bed, equation 1.27 can be transformed to

$$Q = \frac{\Delta PA}{\eta L} \frac{\varepsilon^3}{5(1 - \varepsilon)^2 S_0^2} \tag{1.28}$$

This analysis shows that permeability is a complex function of porosity and surface area, the latter being determined by the size distribution and shape of the particles. The appearance of a specific surface in equation 1.28 offers a method for its measurement and provides the basis of fluid permeation methods of size analysis. The equation is also applied in the studies of filtration.

## 1.15 PUMPS

Equations 1.8 and 1.9 examined the power requirement for driving a liquid through a system against an opposing head. This energy is normally added with a pump. In different processes, the quantities to be delivered, the opposing head, and the nature of the fluid vary widely and many pumps are made to meet these different requirements. Basically, however, pumps can be divided into two main categories: positive displacement pumps, which may be reciprocating or rotary, and impeller pumps. Positive displacement pumps displace a fixed volume of fluid with each stroke or revolution. Impeller pumps, on the other hand, impart high kinetic energy to the fluid that is subsequently converted to pressure energy. The volume discharged depends on the opposing head.

Equipment for pumping gases and liquids is essentially similar. Machines delivering gases are commonly called compressors or blowers. Compressors discharge at relatively high pressures and blowers at relatively low pressures. The lower density and viscosity of gases lead to the use of higher operating speeds and, to minimize leakage, smaller clearance between moving parts.

### 1.15.1 Positive Displacement Pumps

Positive displacement pumps are most commonly used for the discharge of relatively small quantities of fluid against relatively large heads. The small clearance between moving parts precludes the pumping of abrasive slurries.

The single-acting piston pump in Figure 1.13(a) exemplifies the reciprocating pump. The fluid is drawn into a cylinder through an inlet valve by movement of the piston to the right. The stroke in the opposite direction drives fluid through the outlet valve. Leakage past the piston may be prevented by rings or packing. Cessation of pumping on the return stroke is overcome in the double-acting piston pump by utilizing the volume on both sides of the piston. Fluid is drawn in on one side by a stroke that delivers the fluid on the other [Figure 1.13(b)]. In both pumps, delivery fluctuates. Operation, however, is simple and both are efficient under widely varying conditions. The principle is widely used in gas compressors. In pumping liquids, no priming is necessary

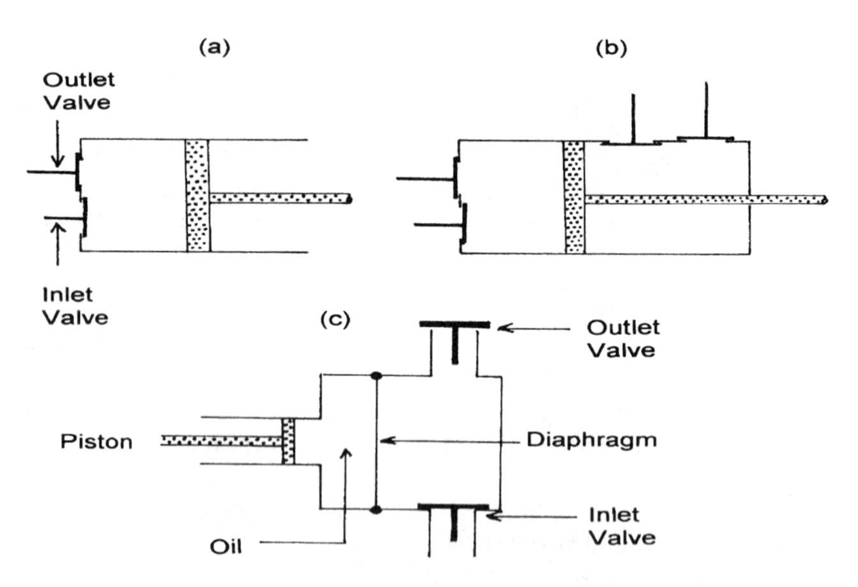


**FIGURE 1.13** Positive displacement pumps.

because the pump will effectively discharge air present in the pump or feed lines.

A modification, known as the diaphragm pump, is constructed so that reciprocating parts do not contact the pumped liquid [Figure 1.13(c)]. A flexible disk, fixed at the periphery, expands and contracts the pumping chamber, drawing in and discharging liquid through valves.

Rotary positive displacement pumps operate by presenting an expanding chamber to the fluid that is then sealed and conveyed to the outlet. Both liquids and gases are discharged so that priming is not necessary. The principle is illustrated in Figure 1.14, which describes a gear pump, a lobe pump, and a vane pump. In the gear pump, the liquid is conveyed in the spaces formed between a case and the consecutive teeth of two gears that intermesh at the center of the pump to prevent return of the liquid to the inlet. The lobe pump, widely used as a liquid pump and as a blower, operates in a similar manner. Each impeller carries two or three lobes that interact with very small clearance to convey fluid from inlet to outlet.

Sliding vanes, mounted in the surface of an off-center rotor but main-

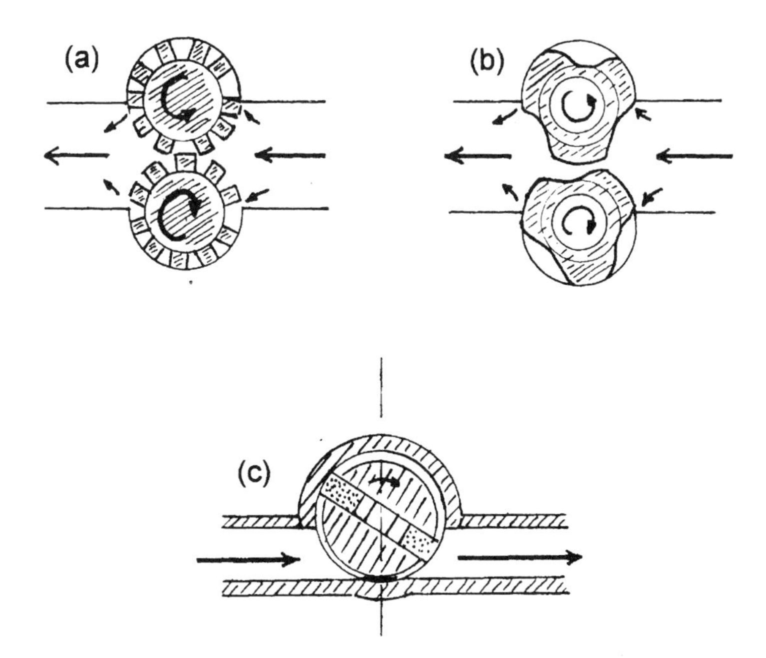


**FIGURE 1.14** Gear, vane, and lobe pumps.

tained in contact with the case by centrifugal force or spring loading, provide the pumping action of the vane pump. Fluid is drawn into the chamber created by two vanes at the inlet. The fluid is rotated and expelled by contraction at the outlet. Besides liquid pumping, the principle of the vane pump is used in blowers and, by evacuating at the inlet and discharging to atmosphere at the outlet, in vacuum pumps.

The Mono pump consists of a stator in the form of a double internal helix and a single helical rotor. The latter maintains a constant seal across the stator and this seal travels continuously through the pump. The pump is suitable for viscous and nonviscous liquids. The stator is commonly made of a rubber or similar material, so slurries are effectively delivered. Discharge is nonpulsating and can be made against very high pressures. The pump is commonly used to drive clarifying and cake filters.

## 1.15.2 Centrifugal Impeller Pumps

The centrifugal impeller pump is the type most widely used in the chemical industry. The impeller consists of a number of vanes, usually curved backward from the direction of rotation. The vanes may be open or, more commonly, closed between one or two supporting plates. This reduces swirl and increases efficiency. The impeller is rotated at high speeds, imparting radial and tangential momenta to a liquid that is fed axially to the center and which spirals through the impeller. In the simple volute pump [Figure 1.15(a)] the liquid is received into a volute chamber. The cross section increases toward the tangential outlet. The liquid therefore decelerates, allowing a conversion of kinetic energy to pressure energy. In the diffuser pump, correctly aligned blades of

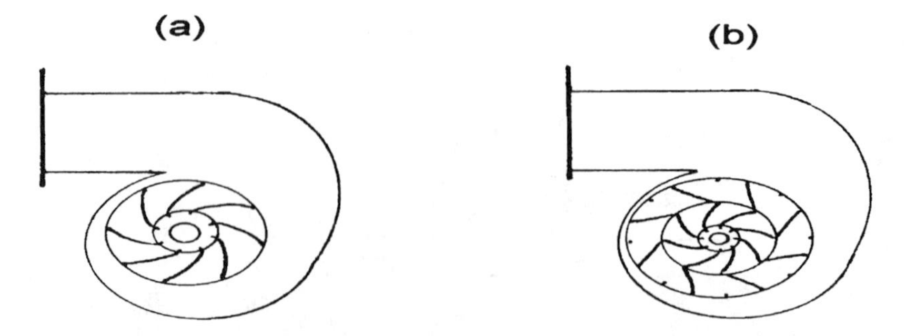


**FIGURE 1.15** Volute pump and diffuser pump.

a diffusing ring over which the fluid velocity decreases smoothly receive the liquid from the impeller and the pressure rises. Flow through a diffuser pump is described in Figure 1.15(b).

Due to the less precise control of the direction of the liquid leaving the impeller, the volute pump is less efficient than the diffuser pump. However, it is more easily fabricated in corrosion-resistant materials and is more commonly used. The pump, which is compact and without valves, may be used to pump slurries and corrosive liquid, steadily delivering large volumes against moderately large heads. For large heads, pumps are used in series. Unlike positive displacement pumps, impeller pumps continue to operate if the delivery line is closed, the kinetic energy of the liquid being degraded to heat.

A disadvantage of the centrifugal pump is that the conditions under which a pump of given size will operate with high efficiency are limited. The relation between the quantity discharged and the opposing head for a volute pump operating at a given speed is shown in Figure 1.16. As the head increases,the quantity discharged decreases. The mechanical efficiency of the pump is the ratio of the power acquired by the liquid, given by equation 1.9, to the power input. A maximum value is shown in Figure 1.16, indicating optimal operating conditions. The effect on the efficiency when the pump operates at other conditions can be seen from the figure, and to achieve reasonable operating efficiency for a given discharge and opposing head a pump of suitable size and operating speed must be used.

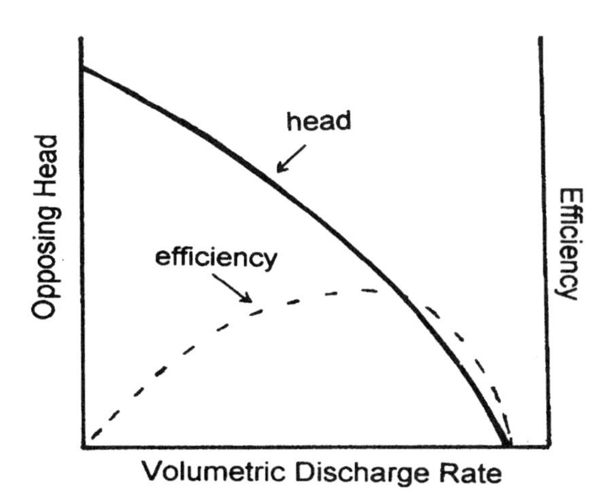


**FIGURE 1.16** Performance curve of a volute pump running at a fixed speed.

A second disadvantage of the centrifugal pump lies in priming. If the pump contains air alone, the low kinetic energy imparted by the impeller creates a very small pressure increase across the pump and liquid is neither drawn into the pump nor discharged. To begin pumping, the impeller must be primed with the liquid to be pumped. Where possible, the pump is placed below the level of the supply. Alternatively, a nonreturn valve could be placed on the suction side of the pump to prevent draining when rotation ceases.

The same principle is employed in centrifugal fans and blowers used to displace large quantities of air and other gases. The gas enters the impeller axially and is moved outward into a scroll. The opposing static head is usually small, and energy appears mainly as the kinetic energy of the moving gas stream.

### 1.15.3 Other Impeller Pumps

The propeller pump, exemplified by a domestic fan, is used to deliver large quantities of fluids against low heads. These conditions are common in recirculation systems. The principle is also employed in fans used for ventilation, the supply of air for drying, and other similar operations.

*Example 1.* In the figure what is the energy loss due to pressure?

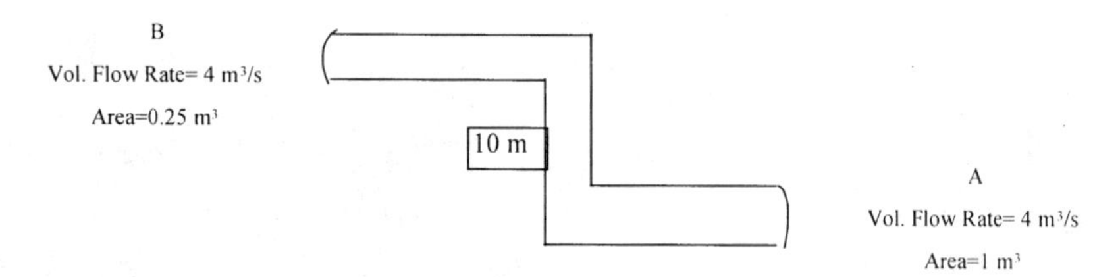


Using Bernoulli's equation, we obtain

$$\frac{u_A^2}{2g} + \frac{P_A}{\rho g} + z_A = \frac{u_B^2}{2g} + \frac{P_B}{\rho g} + z_B + \frac{E}{g}$$

Calculate the velocity head and potential head at points A and B.
Velocity head at A:

$$\frac{\left[\frac{(4\text{m}^3/\text{s})}{(1\text{m}^2)}\right]^2}{2(9.8\text{ m/s}^2)} = 0.82\text{ m}$$

Velocity head at B:

$$\frac{\left[\frac{(4\text{m}^3/\text{s})}{(0.25\text{m}^2)}\right]^2}{2(9.8\ \text{m/s}^2)} = 13\ \text{m}$$

Potential head at A = 0 m
Potential head at B = 10 m
Friction head = 0 m

$$\therefore \quad \frac{P_B - P_A}{\rho g} = 22.18\ \text{m}$$

*Example 2.* Calculation of pressure drop in a pipe due to friction.

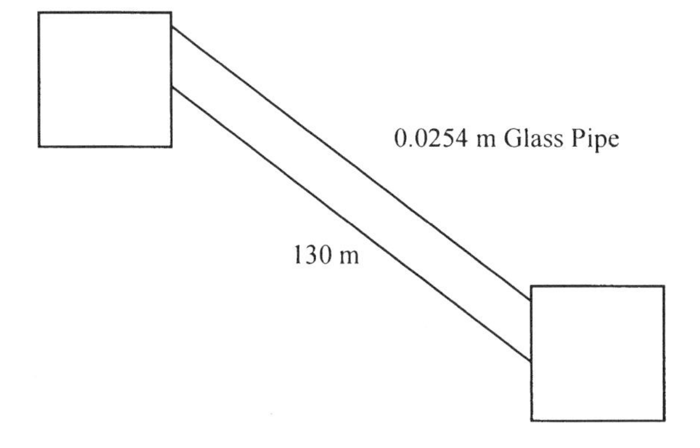


For a smooth 0.08 m pipe, 130 m long, find the friction head. The density of water is 1000 kg/m$^3$, the viscosity of water is $9.28 \times 10^{-5}$ kg-m/s, the mean velocity of flow is 1.8 m/s.

Calculate the Reynolds number.

$$\text{Re} = \frac{(1.8\ \text{m/s})(0.0254\ \text{m})(1000\ \text{kg/m}^3)}{(9.28 \times 10^{-5}\text{lb-ft/s})} = 4.93 \times 10^4$$

$$\frac{R}{\rho u^2} = 2.5 \times 10^{-3}$$

$$R = (2.5 \times 10^{-3})(1000\ \text{kg/m}^3)(1.8\ \text{m/s})^2 = 8.1\ \text{N/m}^2$$

$$\Delta P = \frac{4RL}{d} = \frac{(4)(8.1\ \text{N/m}^2)(130\ \text{m})}{0.0254\ \text{n}} = 1.7 \times 10^5\ \text{N/m}^2$$

$$\text{Friction head} = \frac{1.7 \times 10^5\ \text{N/m}^2}{(1000\ \text{kg/m}^3)(9.8\ \text{m/s}^2)} = 17\ \text{m}$$

# 2

# Heat Transfer

Heat transfer is a major unit operation in pharmacy. Heat energy can only be transferred from a region of higher temperature to a region of lower temperature. Understanding heat transfer requires the study of the mechanism and rate of this process. Heat is transferred by three mechanisms: conduction, convection, and radiation. It is unusual for the transfer to take place by one mechanism only.

*Conduction* is the most widely studied mechanism of heat transfer and the most significant in solids. The flow of heat depends on the transfer of vibrational energy from one molecule to another and, in the case of metals, the movement of free electrons such that no appreciable displacement of matter occurs. Radiation is rare in solids, but examples are found among glasses and plastics. Convection, by definition, is not possible in these conditions. Conduction in the bulk of fluids is normally overshadowed by convection, but it assumes great importance at fluid boundaries.

The motion of fluids transfers heat between the fluids by *convection*. In natural convection the movement is caused by buoyancy forces induced by variations in the density of the fluid, caused by differences in temperature. In forced convection the movement is created by an external energy source, such as a pump.

All bodies with a temperature above absolute zero radiate heat in the form of electromagnetic waves. *Radiation* may be transmitted, reflected, or absorbed by matter, the fraction absorbed being transformed into heat. Radiation is important at extremes of temperature and in circumstances in which the other modes of heat transmission are suppressed. Although heat losses can, in some cases, equal the losses by natural convection, the mechanism is, from the standpoint of pharmaceutical processing, least important and needs only brief consideration.

Heat transfer in many systems occurs as a steady-state process and the temperature at any point in the system will not vary with time. In other important processes, temperatures in the system do vary with time. The latter, which is common among the small-scale, batch-operated processes of the pharmaceutical and fine chemicals industry, is known as unsteady heat transfer, and, since warming or cooling occurs, the thermal capacity (i.e., the size and specific heat) of the system becomes important. Unsteady heat transfer is a complex phenomenon that is difficult to analyze from first principles at a fundamental level.

## 2.1 HEAT TRANSFER BETWEEN FLUIDS

The transfer of heat from one fluid to another across a solid boundary is of great importance in pharmaceutical processing. The system, which frequently varies in nature from one process to another, can be divided into constituent parts and each part characterized in its resistance to the transfer of heat. The whole system may be considered in terms of the equation

$$\text{Rate at which heat is transferred} \propto \frac{\text{Total temperature difference}}{\text{Total thermal resistance}}$$

A hot liquid passing through a heavily lagged metal pipe may be considered as an example. The transfer of heat from the liquid to the pipe, conduction through the pipe wall and across the insulation, and heat loss to the surroundings by natural convection can each be assigned a thermal resistance. A system in which steam is admitted to the outside of a vertical pipe containing a boiling liquid may serve as a second example. This arrangement is common in evaporators, and the evaluation of heat transfer rates demands a study of condensation, conduction across the wall of the tube and any deposited scale, and the mechanism of boiling.

## 2.2 HEAT TRANSFER THROUGH A WALL

Heat transfer by conduction through walls follows the basic relation given by Fourier's equation where the rate of heat flow, $Q$, is proportional to the temperature gradient, $dT/dx$, and to the area normal to the heat flow, $A$:

$$Q = -kA\frac{dT}{dx} \tag{2.1}$$

As the distance, $x$, increases, the temperature, $T$, decreases. Hence, measuring in the $x$ direction, $dT/dx$ is algebraically negative. The proportionality constant $k$ is the thermal conductivity. Its numerical value depends on the material of which the body is made and on its temperature. Values of $k$ for various materials are given in Table 2.1. Metals have high conductivity, although values vary widely. The nonmetallic solids normally have lower conductivities than metals. For the porous materials of this group, the overall conductivity lies between that of the homogeneous solid and the air that permeates the structure. Low resultant values lead to their wide use as heat insulators. Carbon is an exception among nonmetals. Its relatively high conductivity and chemical inertness permit its wide use in heat exchangers.

Steady nondirectional heat transfer through a plane wall of thickness $x$ and area $A$ is represented in Figure 2.1(a). If the thermal conductivity does not change with temperature, the temperature gradient is linear and equal to $(T_1 - T_2)/x$, where $T_1$ is the temperature of the hot face and $T_2$ is the temperature of the cool face. Equation 2.1 then becomes

$$Q = kA\frac{T_1 - T_2}{x} \tag{2.2}$$

which may be rearranged to

$$Q = A\frac{T_1 - T_2}{x} \tag{2.3}$$

where $x/k$ is the thermal resistance. Thus, for a given heat flow, a large temperature drop must be created if the wall or layer has a high thermal resistance. An increase in thermal resistance will reduce the heat flow promoted by a given temperature difference. This is the principle of insulation by lagging,

**TABLE 2.1** Thermal Conductivity, $k$, of Various Materials in J/s-m-K

| Solids | Temp. K | $k$ | Liquids | Temp. K | $k$ | Gases | Temp. K | $k$ |
|---|---|---|---|---|---|---|---|---|
| *Metals* | | | Mercury | 273 | 8.3 | Air | 473 | 0.0311 |
| Copper | 373 | 379 | Acetone | 313 | 0.17 | Steam | 373 | 0.0235 |
| Silver | 373 | 410 | Water | 373 | 0.67 | Carbon dioxide | 373 | 0.022 |
| Cast iron | 373 | 46.4 | | | | Hydrogen | 373 | 0.215 |
| Stainless steel | 373 | 17.3 | | | | | | |
| *Nonmetals* | | | | | | | | |
| Carbon (graphite) | 323 | 138.4 | | | | | | |
| Glass | 373 | 1.16 | | | | | | |
| Building brick | 293 | 0.66 | | | | | | |
| Glass wool | 373 | 0.062 | | | | | | |

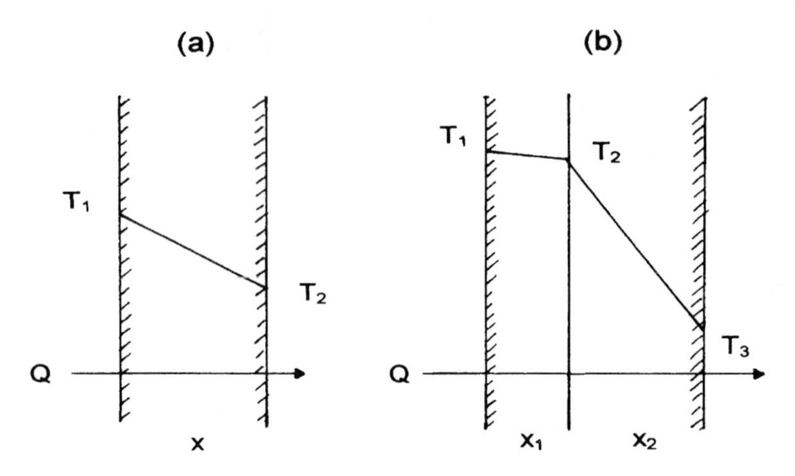


**FIGURE 2.1** Conduction of heat through a wall.

and it is illustrated by a composite wall in Figure 2.1(b). The rate of heat transfer is the same for both materials if steady-state heat transfer exists. Therefore,

$$Q = \frac{k_1 A(T_1 - T_2)}{x_1} = \frac{k_2 A(T_2 - T_3)}{x_2}$$

The major temperature drop occurs across the distance $x_2$ since this material provides the major thermal resistance. (In the case of heavily lagged, thin metal walls, the temperature drop and thermal resistance of the metal are so small that they can be ignored.) Rearranging this equation and eliminating the junction temperature give

$$Q = A \frac{T_1 - T_3}{x_1/k_1 + x_2/k_2} \tag{2.4}$$

Equations of this form can be applied to any number of layers.

## 2.3 HEAT TRANSFER IN PIPES AND TUBES

Pipes and tubes are common barriers over which heat exchange takes place. Conduction is complicated in this case by the changing area over which heat is transferred. If equation 2.2 is to be retained, some value of $A$ must be derived from the length of the pipe, $l$, and the internal and external radii, $r_1$ and $r_2$, respectively. When the pipe is thin-walled and $r_2/r_1 \lesssim 1.5$, the heat transfer area can be based on an arithmetic mean of the two radii. Equation 2.2 then becomes

$$Q = k2\pi\frac{r_2 + r_1}{2}l\frac{T_1 - T_2}{r_2 - r_1} \tag{2.5}$$

This equation is inaccurate for thick-walled pipes. Heat transfer area must then be calculated from the logarithmic mean radius, $r_m$. The equation for heat transfer is then

$$Q = k2\pi r_m l\frac{T_1 - T_2}{r_2 - r_1} \tag{2.6}$$

where

$$r_m = \frac{r_2 - r_1}{\log_e(r_2/r_1)}$$

## 2.4 HEAT EXCHANGE BETWEEN A FLUID AND A SOLID BOUNDARY

Conduction and convection contribute to the transfer of heat from a fluid to a boundary. The distribution of temperatures at a plane barrier separating two fluids is shown in Figure 2.2. If the fluids are in turbulent motion, temperature

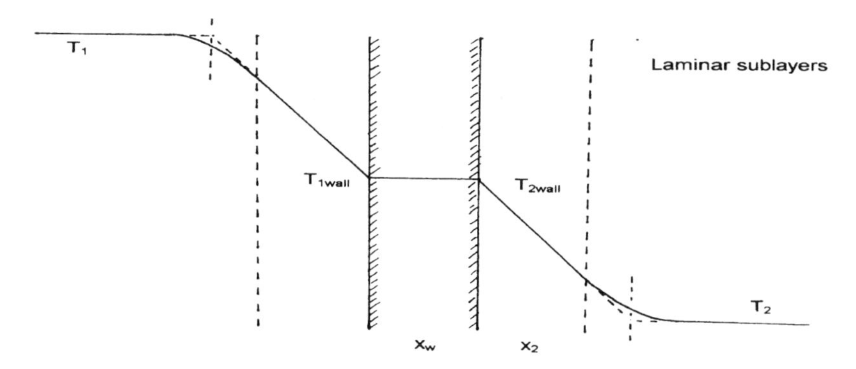


**FIGURE 2.2** Heat transfer between fluids.

gradients are confined to a relatively narrow region adjacent to the wall. Outside this region, turbulent mixing, the mechanism of which is explained in Chapter 1, is very effective in the transfer of heat. Temperature gradients are quickly destroyed, and equalization of values $T_1$ and $T_2$ occurs. Within the region, there exists a laminar sublayer across which heat is transferred by conduction only. Reference to Table 2.1 shows that the thermal conductivity of most fluids is small. The temperature gradients produced by a given heat flow are correspondingly high. Outside the laminar layer, eddies contribute to the transfer of heat by moving fluid from the turbulent bulk to the edge of the sublayer, where heat can be lost or gained, and by corresponding movements in the opposite direction. The temperature gradients in this region, where both convection and conduction contribute to heat transfer, are smaller than in the sublayer.

The major resistance to heat flow resides in the laminar sublayer. Its thickness, therefore, is of critical importance in determining the rate of heat transfer from the fluid to the boundary. The thickness depends on the physical properties of the fluid, the flow conditions, and the nature of the surface. Increase in flow velocity, for example, decreases the thickness of the layer and, therefore, its resistance to heat flow. The interaction of these variables is exceedingly complex.

A film, transmitting heat only by conduction, may be postulated in order to evaluate the rate of heat transfer at a boundary. This fictitious film presents the same resistance to heat transfer as the complex turbulent and laminar regions near the wall. If, on the hot side of the wall, the fictitious layer had a thickness $x_1$, the equation of heat transfer to the wall would be

$$Q = kA\,\frac{(T_1 - T_{1\text{wall}})}{x_1}$$

where $k$ is the thermal conductivity of the fluid. A similar equation applies to heat transfer at the cold side of the wall. The layer thickness is determined by the same factors that control the extent of the laminar sublayer. In general it is not known, and the previous equation may be rewritten

$$Q = h_1 A(T_1 - T_{1\text{wall}}) \qquad (2.7)$$

where $h_1$ is the heat transfer coefficient for the film under discussion. It corresponds to the ratio $k/x_1$ and has units J/m$^2$-s K. This is a convenient, numerical expression of the flow of heat by conduction and convection at a boundary. Typical values of heat transfer or film coefficients are given in Table 2.2. The approximate evaluation of these coefficients is discussed in the next section.

**TABLE 2.2** Film Coefficient $h$ for Various Fluids (J/m$^2$-s-K)

| Fluid | $h$ |
|---|---|
| Water | 1700–11350 |
| Gases | 17–285 |
| Organic solvents | 340–2840 |
| Oils | 57–680 |

The ratio of the temperature difference and the total thermal resistance determines the rate of heat transfer across the three layers of Figure 2.2. Using the film coefficient $h_2$ to characterize heat transfer from the barrier to the colder fluid, one obtains

$$T_1 - T_{1\text{wall}} = \frac{Q}{h_1 A}$$

$$T_{1\text{wall}} - T_{2\text{wall}} = \frac{Q x_w}{k_w A}$$

where $k_w$ is the thermal conductivity of the wall.

$$T_{2\text{wall}} - T_2 = \frac{Q}{h_2 A}$$

Adding and rearranging these equations give

$$Q = \frac{A}{1/h_1 + x_w/k_w + 1/h_2}(T_1 - T_2) \tag{2.8}$$

The quantity

$$\frac{1}{1/h_1 + x_w/k_w + 1/h_2}$$

is called the overall heat transfer coefficient, $U$. A general expression of the rate of heat transfer then becomes

$$Q = UA\Delta T \tag{2.9}$$

## 2.5 APPLICATION OF DIMENSIONAL ANALYSIS TO CONVECTIVE HEAT TRANSFER

Dimensional analysis offers a rational approach to the estimation of the complex phenomena of convective heat transfer rates.

Free convection describes heat transfer by the bulk movement of fluids induced by buoyancy forces. These arise from the variation of fluid density with temperature. If the surface in contact with the fluid is hotter, the fluid will absorb heat, a local decrease in density will occur, and some of the fluid will rise. If the surface is colder, the reverse takes place. For these conditions, the following factors will influence the heat transferred per unit area per unit time, $q$. The dimensional form of these factors is given, using the additional fundamental dimensions of temperature, [θ], and heat [H]. The latter is justified if interchange of heat energy and mechanical energy is precluded. This is approximately true in the subject under discussion, the heat produced by frictional effects, for example, being negligible.

| | |
|---|---|
| The viscosity of the fluid, $\eta$. | $[\mathrm{M\,L^{-1}\,T^{-1}}]$ |
| The thermal conductivity of the fluid, $k$. | $[\mathrm{H\,T^{-1}\,L^{-1}\,\theta^{-1}}]$ |
| The temperature difference between the surface and the bulk of the fluid, $\Delta T$. | $[\theta]$ |
| The density, $\rho$. | $[\mathrm{M\,L^{-3}}]$ |
| The specific heat, $C_p$. | $[\mathrm{H\,M^{-1}\,\theta^{-1}}]$ |
| The buoyancy forces. They depend on the product of the coefficient of thermal expansion $a$, and the acceleration due to gravity, $g$. | $[\theta^{-1}\,\mathrm{L\,T^{-2}}]$ |

Normally only one dimension, that of the physical dimensions of the surface, is important. For example, the height of a plane vertical surface has greater significance than the width that only determined the total area involved. The important characteristic dimension is designated $l$ [L]. The equation of dimensions is then

$$[q] = [l^x \Delta T^y k^z \eta^p C_p^q (ag)^r \rho^s]$$

or

$$[\mathrm{H\,L^{-2}\,T^{-1}}] = [\mathrm{L}^x\theta^y\mathrm{H}^z\mathrm{T}^{-z}\mathrm{L}^{-z}\theta^{-z}\mathrm{M}^p\mathrm{L}^{-p}\mathrm{T}^{-p}\mathrm{H}^q\mathrm{M}^{-q}\theta^{-q}\theta^{-r}\mathrm{L}^r\mathrm{T}^{-2r}\mathrm{M}^s\mathrm{L}^{-3s}]$$

Equating indices gives

$$\mathrm{H} \qquad 1 = q + z$$

$$\mathrm{L} \qquad -2 = x - p + r - 3s - z$$

$$\begin{array}{ll} \text{T} & -1 = -p - 2r - z \\ \theta & \quad 0 = y - q - r - z \\ \text{M} & \quad 0 = p - q + s \end{array}$$

Solving for $x$, $y$, $z$, $p$, and $s$ in terms of $q$ and $r$ gives

$$\begin{aligned} z &= 1 - q \\ y &= r + 1 \\ p &= q - 2r \\ s &= 2r \\ x &= 3r - 1 \end{aligned}$$

Therefore,

$$[q] = [l^{3r-1}\,\Delta T^{r+1} C_p^q k^{1-q} (ag)^r \rho^{2r} \eta^{q-2}]$$

Collecting into three groups the variables to the power of 1, the power $q$, and the power $r$, we can write

$$q = \text{Constant}\,\frac{\Delta Tk}{l}\left(\frac{l^3 \Delta T a g \rho^2}{\eta^2}\right)^r \left(\frac{C_p\,\eta}{k}\right)^q$$

or

$$\frac{ql}{\Delta Tk} = \text{Constant}\left(\frac{l^3 \Delta T a g \rho^2}{\eta^2}\right)^r \left(\frac{C_p \eta}{k}\right)^q \tag{2.10}$$

Heat transfer by free convection can thus be presented as a relation between three dimensionless groups. The quantity $C_p\eta/k$ is known as the Prandtl number, the combination $l^3\Delta T a g\rho^2/\eta^2$ is known as the Grashof number, and $ql/\Delta Tk$ is the Nusselt number. Since the film coefficient, $h$, is given by $q/\Delta T$, the Nusselt number may also be written $hl/k$.

The specific relation in which these groups stand is established for a particular system by experiment. Then, for the same geometric arrangement, in which heat is transferred by free convection, the correlation allows the Nusselt number, Nu, to be determined with reasonable accuracy from known values of the variables which constitute the Grashof number, Gr, and the Prandtl number, Pr. From Nu, the heat transferred per unit area per unit time, $q$, and the film coefficient, $h$, can be determined.

The fluid properties $C_p$, $k$, $\eta$, and $\rho$ are themselves temperature dependent. In establishing a correlation, the temperature at which these properties are to be measured must be chosen. This temperature is usually that of the main body of the fluid or the mean of this temperature and the surface temperature.

Experimental correlations for many surface configurations are available. The exponents $r$ and $q$ are usually equal to 0.25 in streamline flow and 0.33 in turbulent flow. The constant varies with the physical configuration. As an example, the heat transfer to gases and liquids from a large horizontal pipe by free convection is described by the relation

$$\frac{qd}{k\Delta T} = 0.47\left(\frac{d^3\ \Delta Tag\rho^2}{\eta^2}\right)^{0.25}\left(\frac{C_p\eta}{k}\right)^{0.25} \tag{2.11}$$

The linear dimension in this correlation is the pipe diameter $d$. The fluid properties are to be measured at the mean of the wall and bulk fluid temperatures.

In forced convection the fluid is moved over the surface by a pump or blower. The effects of natural convection are usually neglected. The study of forced convection is of great practical importance, and a vast amount of data has been documented for streamline and turbulent flows in pipes, across and parallel to tubes, across plane surfaces, and in other important configurations such as jackets and coils. Such data is again correlated by means of dimensionless groups.

In forced convection the heat transferred per unit area per unit time, $q$, is determined by a linear dimension which characterizes the surface, $l$, the temperature difference between the surface and the fluid, $\Delta T$, the viscosity, $\eta$, density, $\rho$, and velocity, $u$, of the fluid, its conductivity, $k$, and its specific heat, $C_p$. Dimensional analysis yields the relation

$$\frac{ql}{k\Delta T} = \text{Constant}\left(\frac{C_p\eta}{k}\right)^x\left(\frac{ul\rho}{\eta}\right)^y \tag{2.12}$$

where $ql/k\Delta T$ is the Nusselt number, Nu, $C_p\eta/k$ is the Prandtl number, Pr, and $ul\rho/\eta$ is Reynolds number, Re, a parameter discussed in Chapter 1. The values of the indices $x$ and $y$ and of the constant are established for a particular system by experiment. For turbulent flow in pipes, the correlation for fluids of low viscosity is

$$\mathrm{Nu} = 0.023\ \mathrm{Pr}^x\ \mathrm{Re}^{0.8} \tag{2.13}$$

where $x = 0.4$ for heating and 0.3 for cooling. The linear dimension used to calculate Re or Nu is the pipe diameter, and the physical properties of the fluid are to be measured at the bulk fluid temperature. This relation shows that in a given system, the film coefficient varies as the fluid velocity$^{0.8}$. If the flow velocity is doubled, the film coefficient increases by a factor of 1.7.

Although the correlations given may appear complex, their use in practice is often simple. A large quantity of tabulated data is available, and numerical values of the variables and their dimensionless combinations are readily accessible. The graphical presentation of these variables or groups in many cases permits an easy solution. In other cases the correlation can be greatly simplified if it is restricted to a particular system. Free convection to air is an important example.

## 2.6 HEAT TRANSFER TO BOILING LIQUIDS

Heat transfer to boiling liquids occurs in several operations, such as distillation and evaporation. Heat is transferred by conduction and convection in a process further complicated by the change of phase which occurs at the heating boundary. When boiling is induced by a heater in contact with a pool of liquid, the process is known as pool boiling. Liquid movement is derived only from heating effects. In other systems, the boiling liquid may be driven through or over heaters, a process referred to as boiling with forced circulation.

## 2.7 POOL BOILING

If a horizontal heating surface is in contact with a boiling liquid, a sequence of events occurs as the temperature difference between the surface and the liquid increases. Figure 2.3 relates heat flux per unit area at the surface, $q$, to the temperature difference between the surface and boiling water, $\Delta T$. The derived value of the heat transfer coefficient, $h = q/\Delta T$, is also plotted.

When $\Delta T$ is small, the degree of superheating of the liquid layers adjacent to the surface is low, and bubble formation, growth, and disengagement, if present, are slow. Liquid disturbance is small, and heat transfer can be estimated from expressions for natural convection given, for example, in equation

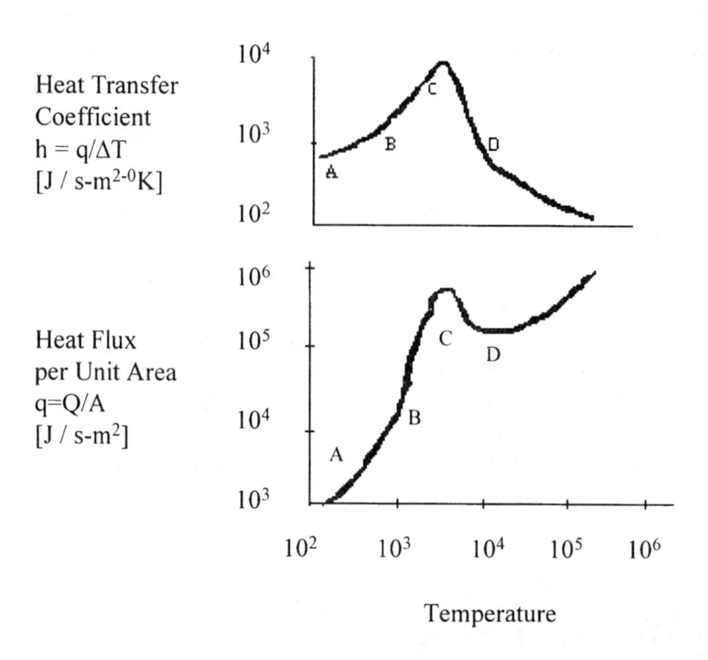


**FIGURE 2.3** Variation in heat transfer coefficient and heat flux per unit area.

2.11. This regime corresponds to section AB of Figure 2.3, over which both $q$ and $h$ increase.

In section BC, vapor formation becomes more vigorous, and bubble chains rise from points which progressively increase in number and finally merge. This movement increases liquid circulation and $q$ and $h$ rise rapidly. This phase is called nucleate boiling and is the practically important regime. For water, approximate values of $q$ and $h$ may be read from Figure 2.3. At point C a peak flux occurs and a maximum heat transfer coefficient is obtained. At this point $\Delta T$ is known as the critical temperature drop. For water, the value lies between 25 and 32 K. The critical temperature drop for organic liquids is somewhat higher. Beyond C, vapor formation is so rapid that escape is inadequate and a progressively larger fraction of the heating surface becomes covered with a vapor film, the low conductivity of which leads to a decrease in $q$ and $h$. This represents a transition from nucleate boiling to film boiling. When this transition is complete (D), the vapor entirely covers the surface, film boiling is fully established, and the heat flux again rises.

The low heat transfer coefficient renders film boiling undesirable, and equipment is designed for and operated at temperature differences that are less than the critical temperature drop. If a constant temperature heat source, such as steam or hot liquid, is employed, exceeding the critical temperature drop results simply in a drop in heat flux and process efficiency. If, however, a constant heat input source is used, as in electrical heating, decreasing heat flux as the transition region is entered causes a sudden and possibly damaging increase in the temperature of the heating element. Damage is known as boiling burnout. Under these circumstances, the region CD of Figure 2.3 is not obtained.

Boiling heat transfer coefficients depend on the physical character of the liquid and the nature of the heating surface. Through the agencies of wetting, roughness, and contamination, the latter greatly influences the formation, growth, and disengagement of bubbles in the nucleate boiling regime. At present there is no reliable method of estimating the boiling coefficients of heat transfer from the physical properties of the system. Coefficients, as shown for water in Figure 2.3, are large, and higher resistances elsewhere often limit the rate at which heat can be transferred through a system as a whole.

## 2.8 BOILING INSIDE A VERTICAL TUBE

Heat transfer to liquids boiling in vertical tubes is common in evaporators. If a long tube of suitable diameter, in which liquid lies at a low level, is heated, the pattern of boiling shown in Figure 2.4 is established (McCabe et al, 1993). At low levels, boiling may be suppressed by the imposed head [Figure 2.4(a)]. Higher in the tube, bubbles are produced which rise and coalesce [Figure 2.4(b)]. Slug formation due to bubble coagulation occurs [Figure 2.4(c), (d)]. The slugs finally break down [Figure 2.4(e)]. Escape is hindered and both liquid and vapor move upward at increasing speed. Draining leads to separation of the phases, giving an annular film of liquid dragged upward by a core of high-velocity vapor [Figure 2.4(f)]. In long tubes the main heat transfer takes place in this region by forced convection or nucleate boiling. At low temperature differences between wall and film, heat transfer occurs quietly as in forced convection. This is the normal regime in a climbing film evaporator, and heat flux can be calculated from correlations of the type given in equation 2.12. At higher temperature differences, nucleate boiling takes place in the film and the vigorous movement leads to an increase in heat transfer coefficient.

## 2.9 BOILING WITH FORCED CIRCULATION

In many systems, movements other than those caused by boiling are imposed. For example, boiling in agitated vessels is common in many batch processes.

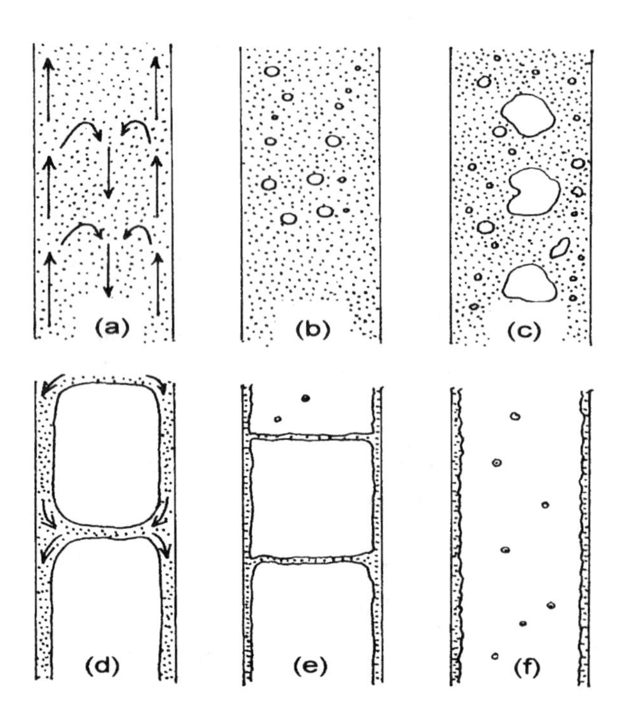


**FIGURE 2.4** Boiling in narrow vertical tube.

The boiling heat transfer coefficients depend on the properties of the liquid, the nature of the surface, and the agitation used. Coefficients obtained are slightly higher than those of pool boiling. Inside tubes the pattern of forced circulation boiling is similar to that described in the previous section. Coefficients, however, are higher because the velocities attained are higher.

## 2.10 HEAT TRANSFER FROM CONDENSING VAPORS

When a saturated vapor is brought into contact with a cool surface, heat is transferred to the surface and a liquid condenses. The vapor may consist of a single substance or a mixture, some components of which may be noncondensable. The process is described by the following sequence: The vapor diffuses to the boundary where actual condensation takes place. In most cases, the condensate forms a continuous layer over the cooling surface, draining under the influence of gravity. This process is known as film condensation. The latent heat liberated is transferred through the film to the surface by conduction. Although this film offers considerable resistance to heat flow, film coefficients are usually high.

## 2.11 DROPWISE CONDENSATION

Under some surface conditions the condensate does not form a continuous film. Droplets are formed which grow, coalesce, and then run from the surface. Since a fraction of the surface is always directly exposed to the vapor, film resistance is absent and heat transfer coefficients that may be 10 times those of film condensation are obtained. This process is known as dropwise condensation. Although highly desirable, its occurrence, which depends on the wettability of the surface, is not predictable and cannot be used as a basis for design.

## 2.12 CONDENSATION OF A PURE VAPOR

For film condensation a theoretical analysis of the laminar flow of a liquid film down an inclined surface and the progressive increase in thickness due to condensation yields the following expression for the mean heat transfer coefficient, $h_m$:

$$h_m = \text{Constant}\left(\frac{\rho^2 k^3 \lambda g}{\Delta T \eta x}\right)^{0.25} \tag{2.14}$$

where $\lambda$ is the latent heat of vaporization, and $\rho$, $k$, and $\eta$ are the liquid's density, thermal conductivity, and viscosity, respectively; $\Delta T$ is the difference in temperature between the surface and the vapor. Experimentally determined coefficients confirm the validity of equation 2.14. In practice, however, coefficients are somewhat higher due to disturbance of the film arising from a number of factors. As the condensation rate rises, the thickness of the condensate layer increases and the film coefficient falls. However, a point may be reached in long vertical tubes at which flow in the layer becomes turbulent. Under these conditions the coefficient again rises, and equation 2.14 is not valid. Coefficients may also be increased if high vapor velocities induce ripples in the film.

## 2.13 CONDENSATION OF MIXED VAPORS

If a mixture of condensable and noncondensable gases is cooled below its dew point at a surface, the former condenses leaving the adjacent layers richer in the latter, thus creating an added thermal resistance. The condensable fraction must diffuse through this layer to reach the film of condensate, and heat transfer coefficients are normally very much lower than the corresponding value for the pure vapor. For example, the presence of 0.5% of air has been found to reduce the heat transfer by condensation of steam by as much as 50%.

## 2.14 HEAT TRANSFER BY RADIATION

There is continuous interchange of energy between bodies by the emission and absorption of radiation. If two adjacent surfaces are at different temperatures, the hotter surface radiates more energy than it receives and its temperature falls. The cooler surface receives more energy than it emits and its temperature rises. Ultimately thermal equilibrium is reached. Interchange of energy continues but gains and losses are equal.

Of the radiation which falls on a body, a fraction, $a$, is absorbed, a fraction, $r$, is reflected, and a fraction, $t$, is transmitted. These fractions are called the *absorptivity*, the *reflectivity*, and the *transmissivity*, respectively. Most industrial solids are opaque, so the transmissivity is zero and

$$a + r = 1 \tag{2.15}$$

Reflectivity and, therefore, absorptivity depend greatly on the nature of the surface. The limiting case—that of a body which absorbs all and reflects none of the incident radiation—is called a blackbody.

## 2.15 EXCHANGE OF RADIATION

The exchange of radiation is based on two laws. The first, known as Kirchhoff's law, states that the ratio of the emissive power to the absorptivity is the same for all bodies in thermal equilibrium. The emissive power of a body, $E$, is the radiant energy emitted from unit area in unit time (J/m$^2$-s). A body of area $A_1$ and emissivity $E_1$ therefore emits energy at a rate $E_1A_1$. If the radiation falling on unit area of the body is $E_b$, the rate of energy absorption is $E_ba_1A_1$, where $a_1$ is the absorptivity. At thermal equilibrium, $E_ba_1A_1 = E_1A_1$. For another body in the same environment, $E_ba_2A_2 = E_2A_2$. Therefore,

$$E_h = \frac{E_1}{a_1} = \frac{E_2}{a_2} \tag{2.16}$$

For a blackbody, $a = 1$. The emissive power is therefore $E_b$. The blackbody is a perfect radiator and is used as the comparative standard for other surfaces. The *emissivity* of a surface is defined as the ratio of the emissive power, $E$, of the surface to the emissive power of a blackbody at the same temperature, $E_b$:

$$e = \frac{E}{E_b} \tag{2.17}$$

The emissivity is numerically equal to the absorptivity. Since the emissive power varies with wavelength, the ratio should be quoted at a particular wavelength. For many materials, however, the emissive power is a constant fraction of the blackbody radiation; i.e., the emissivity is constant. These materials are known as graybodies.

The second fundamental law of radiation, known as the Stefan-Boltzmann law, states that the rate of energy emission from a blackbody is proportional to the fourth power of the absolute temperature, $T$:

$$E = \sigma T^4 \tag{2.18}$$

where $E$ is the total emissive power and $\sigma$ is the Stefan-Boltzmann constant, the numerical value of which is $5.676 \times 10^{-8}$ J/m$^2$-s-K$^4$. It is sufficiently accurate to say that the heat emitted in unit time, $Q$, from a blackbody of area $A$ is

$$Q = \sigma A T^4$$

and for a body which is not perfectly black by

$$Q = \sigma e A T^4 \tag{2.19}$$

where $e$ is the emissivity.

The net energy gained or lost by a body can be estimated with these laws. The simplest case is that of a graybody in black surroundings. These conditions, in which none of the energy emitted by the body is reflected back, are approximately those of a body radiating to atmosphere. If the absolute temperature of the body is $T_1$, the rate of heat loss is $\sigma e A T_1^4$ (equation 2.19), where $A$ is the area of the body and $e$ is its emissivity. Surroundings at a temperature $T_2$ will emit radiation proportional to $\sigma T_2^4$ and a fraction, determined by area and absorptivity, $a$, will be absorbed by the body. This heat will be $\sigma a A T_2^4$, and since absorptivity and emissivity are equal

$$\text{Net heat transfer rate} = \sigma e A(T_1^4 - T_2^4) \quad (2.20)$$

If part of the energy emitted by a surface is reflected back by another surface, the calculation of radiation exchange is more complex. Equations for various surface configurations are available. These take the general form

$$Q = F_1 F_2 \sigma A(T_A^4 - T_B^4)$$

where $F_1$ and $F_2$ are factors determined by the configuration and emissivity of surfaces at temperatures $T_A$ and $T_B$.

*Example 1.* A stainless steel pipe has an internal radius of 0.019 m and an external radius of 0.024 m. The thermal conductivity of stainless steel is 34.606 J/m-s-K. Steam at 422 K surrounds the pipe, which is lagged with 0.051 m of insulation with a conductivity of 0.069 J/m-s-K. The temperature of the outer surface of the insulation is 311 K. What is the heat loss per meter of pipe?

For the wall of the pipe,

$$\frac{0.024 \text{ m}}{0.019 \text{ m}} = 1.3 < 1.5$$

Therefore, the arithmetic mean best defines the radius:

$$r = \frac{0.019 \text{ m} + 0.024 \text{ m}}{2} = 0.022 \text{ m}$$

For the insulation,

$$\frac{0.051 \text{ m}}{0.024 \text{ m}} = 2.1 > 1.5$$

Therefore, the logarithmic mean best defines the radius:

$$r_m = \frac{0.051 - 0.024}{2.3\log(0.051/0.024)} = 0.036 \text{ m}$$

For the pipe,

$$Q = (34.606 \text{ J/m-s-K})(2\pi)(0.022 \text{ m})(1 \text{ m})\left(\frac{T_1 - T_2}{0.024 \text{ m} - 0.019 \text{ m}}\right)$$

$$= 957(T_1 - T_2)$$

For the insulation,

$$Q = (0.069 \text{ J/m-s-K})(2\,\pi)(0.036 \text{ m})(1 \text{ m})\left(\frac{T_2 - T_3}{0.051 \text{ m} - 0.024 \text{ m}}\right)$$

$$= 0.578(T_2 - T_3)$$

Rearranging these equations gives

$$T_1 - T_2 = \frac{Q}{957} \qquad T_2 - T_3 = \frac{Q}{0.578}$$

Thus,

$$T_1 - T_3 = 111 \text{ K} = \frac{Q}{957} + \frac{Q}{0.578}$$

and

$$Q = \frac{111}{1/957 + 1/0.578} = 64 \text{ J/s}$$

*Example 2.* A 0.051-m uninsulated horizontal pipe is carrying steam at 389 K to the surroundings at 294 K. The emissivity, $e$, of the pipe is 0.8. Absolute zero is 273 K. Find the heat loss by radiation.

$$\frac{\text{Heat loss}}{\text{Unit length}} =$$

$$(5.676 \times 10^{-8} \text{ J/m}^2\text{-s-K}^4)(0.058 \text{ m})(\pi)(0.8)[(116 \text{ K})^4 - (21 \text{ K})^4]$$

$$= 1.50 \text{ J/m-s}$$

# 3

# Mass Transfer

This chapter briefly reviews mass transfer to complete the overview of the fundamental unit processes in pharmacy. Mass transfer is conceptually and mathematically analogous to heat transfer, as will be seen in the following exposition. Many processes are adopted so that a mixture of materials can be separated into component parts. In some, purely mechanical means are used. Solids may be separated from liquids by the arrest of the former in a bed permeable to the fluid. This process is known as filtration. In other examples, a difference in density of two phases permits separation. This is found in sedimentation and centrifugation. Many other processes, however, operate by a change in the composition of a phase due to the diffusion of one component in another. Such processes are known as diffusional or mass transfer processes. Distillation, dissolution, drying, and crystallization are examples of mass transfer processes. In all cases, diffusion is the result of a difference in the concentration of the diffusing substance. This component moves from a region of high concentration to a region of low concentration under the influence of the concentration gradient.

In mass transfer operations, two immiscible phases are normally present, one or both of which are fluid. In general, these phases are in relative motion and the rate at which a component is transferred from one phase to the other is greatly influenced by the bulk movement of the fluids. In most drying processes, for example, water vapor diffuses from a saturated layer in contact with the drying surface into a turbulent airstream. The boundary layer, as described in Chapter 1, consists of a sublayer in which flow is laminar and an outer region in which flow is turbulent. The mechanism of diffusion differs in these regimes. In the laminar layer, movement of water vapor molecules across streamlines can only occur by molecular diffusion. In the turbulent region the movement of relatively large units of gas, called eddies, from one region to another causes mixing of the gas components. This mixing is called eddy diffusion. Eddy diffusion is a more rapid process, and although molecular diffusion is still present, its contribution to the overall movement of material is small. In still air, eddy diffusion is virtually absent and evaporation occurs only by molecular diffusion.

## 3.1 MOLECULAR DIFFUSION IN GASES

Transport of material in stagnant fluids or across the streamlines of a fluid in laminar flow occurs by molecular diffusion. In Figure 3.1, two adjacent compartments, separated by a partition, are drawn. Each compartment contains a pure gas, A or B. Random movement of all molecules occurs so that after a period of time, molecules are found quite remote from their original positions. If the partition is removed, some molecules of A will move toward the

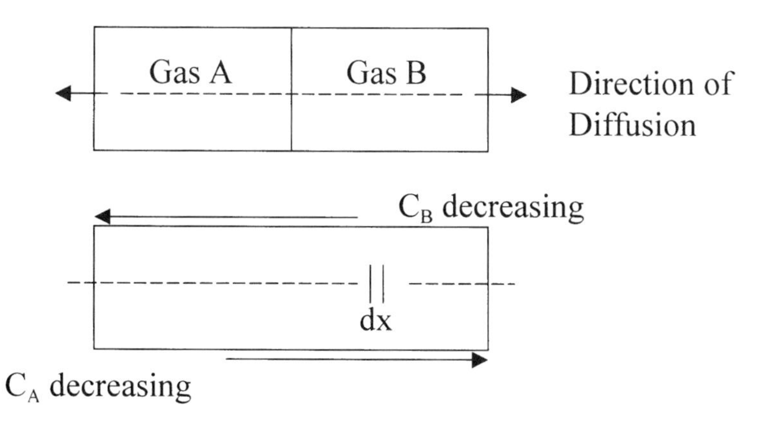


**FIGURE 3.1** Molecular diffusion of gases A and B.

region occupied by B, their number depending on the number of molecules at the point considered. Concurrently, molecules of B diffuse toward regions formerly occupied by pure A. Ultimately, complete mixing occurs. Before this point in time, a gradual variation in the concentration of A exists along an axis, designated $x$, which joins the original compartments. This variation, expressed mathematically, is $-dC_A/dx$, where $C_A$ is the concentration of A. The negative sign arises because the concentration of A decreases as the distance $x$ increases. Similarly, the variation in the concentration of gas B is $-dC_B/dx$. These expressions, which describe the change in the number of molecules of A or B over some small distance in the direction indicated, are concentration gradients. The rate of diffusion of A, $N_A$, depends on the concentration gradient and on the average velocity with which the molecules of A move in the $x$ direction. Fick's law expresses this relationship:

$$N_A = -D_{AB} \frac{dC_A}{dx} \tag{3.1}$$

where $D$ is the diffusivity of A in B. It is a property proportional to the average molecular velocity and, therefore, dependent on the temperature and pressure of the gases. The quantity $N_A$ is usually expressed as the number of moles diffusing across unit area in unit time. In the S.I. unit system, which is used frequently for mass transfer, $N_A$ is expressed as moles per square meter per second. The units of diffusivity then become $m^2\ s^{-1}$. As with the basic equations of heat transfer, equation 3.1 indicates that the rate of a process is directly proportional to a driving force, which, in this context, is a concentration gradient.

This basic equation can be applied to a number of situations. If discussion is restricted exclusively to steady-state conditions, in which neither $dC_A/dx$ or $dC_B/dx$ change with time, then equimolecular counterdiffusion is considered first.

## 3.2 EQUIMOLECULAR COUNTERDIFFUSION

If no bulk flow occurs in the element of length $dx$, shown in Figure 3.1, the rates of diffusion of the two gases, A and B, must be equal and opposite:

$$N_A = -N_B$$

The partial pressure of A changes by $dP_A$ over the distance $dx$. Similarly, the partial pressure of B changes by $dP_B$. Since there is no difference in total pressure across the element (no bulk flow), $dP_A/dx$ must equal $-dP_B/dx$. For an ideal gas, the partial pressure is related to the molar concentration by the relation

$$P_A V = n_A RT$$

where $n_A$ is the number of moles of gas A in a volume $V$. Since the molar concentration, $C_A$, is equal to $n_A/V$,

$$P_A = C_A RT$$

Therefore for gas A, equation 3.1 can be written

$$N_A = -\frac{D_{AB}}{RT}\frac{dP_A}{dx} \tag{3.2}$$

where $D_{AB}$ is the diffusivity of A in B. Similarly,

$$N_B = -\frac{D_{BA}}{RT}\frac{dP_B}{dx} = \frac{D_{AB}}{RT}\frac{dP_A}{dx}$$

It therefore follows that $D_{AB} = D_{BA} = D$. If the partial pressure of A at $x_1$ is $P_{A1}$ and at $x_2$ is $P_{A2}$, integration of equation 3.2 gives

$$N_A = -\frac{D}{RT}\frac{P_{A2} - P_{A1}}{x_2 - x_1} \tag{3.3}$$

A similar equation may be derived for the counterdiffusion of gas B.

## 3.3 DIFFUSION THROUGH A STATIONARY, NONDIFFUSING GAS

An important practical case arises when a gas A diffuses through a gas B, there being no overall transport of gas B. It arises, for example, when a vapor formed at a drying surface diffuses into a surrounding gas. At the liquid surface, the partial pressure of A is dictated by the temperature. For water, it would be 12.8 mmHg at 298 K. Some distance away the partial pressure is lower and the concentration gradient causes diffusion of A away from the surface. Similarly, a concentration gradient for B must exist, the concentration being lowest at the surface. Diffusion of this component takes place toward the surface. There is, however, no overall transport of B, so diffusional movement must be balanced by bulk flow away from the surface. The total flow of A is, therefore, the diffusional flow of A plus the transfer of A associated with this bulk movement.

## 3.4 MOLECULAR DIFFUSION IN LIQUIDS

Equations describing molecular diffusion in liquids are similar to those applied to gases. The rate of diffusion of material A in a liquid is given by equation 3.1:

$$N_{\mathrm{A}} = -D\frac{dC_{\mathrm{A}}}{dx}$$

Fick's law for steady-state, equimolal counterdiffusion is then

$$N_{\mathrm{A}} = -D\frac{C_{\mathrm{A2}} - C_{\mathrm{A1}}}{x_2 - x_1} \tag{3.4}$$

where $C_{\mathrm{A2}}$ and $C_{\mathrm{A1}}$ are the molar concentrations at points $x_2$ and $x_1$, respectively.

Equations for diffusion through a layer of stagnant liquid can also be developed. The use of these equations is, however, limited because diffusivity in a liquid varies with concentration. In addition, unless the solutions are very dilute, the total molar concentration varies from point to point. These complications do not arise with diffusion in gases.

Diffusivities in liquids are very much less than diffusivities in gases, commonly by a factor of $10^4$.

## 3.5 MASS TRANSFER IN TURBULENT AND LAMINAR FLOWS

As already explained, movement of molecules across the streamlines of a fluid in laminar flow can only occur by molecular diffusion. If the concentration of a component, A, varies in a direction normal to the streamlines, the molar rate of diffusion is given by equation 3.1.

When a fluid flows over a surface, the surface retards the adjacent fluid region, forming a boundary layer. If flow throughout the fluid is laminar, the equation for molecular diffusion may be used to evaluate the mass transferred across the boundary layer. In most important cases, however, flow in the bulk of the fluid is turbulent. The boundary layer is then considered to consist of three distinct flow regimes. In the region of the boundary layer most distant from the surface, flow is turbulent and mass transfer is the result of the interchange of large portions of the fluid. Mass interchange is rapid and concentration gradients are low. As the surface is approached, a transition from turbulent flow to laminar flow occurs in the transition or buffer region. In this region, mass transfer by eddy diffusion and molecular diffusion is of comparable magnitude. In a fluid layer at the surface, a fraction of a millimeter thick, laminar flow conditions persist. This laminar sublayer, in which transfer occurs by molecular diffusion only, offers the main resistance to mass transfer, as shown in Figure 3.2. As flow becomes more turbulent, the thickness of the laminar sublayer and its resistance to mass transfer decrease.

One approach to the evaluation of the rate of mass transfer under these conditions lies in the postulation of a film, the thickness of which offers the same resistance to mass transfer as the combined laminar, transition, and turbulent regions. The analogy with heat transfer by conduction and convection is exact, and quantitative relations between heat and mass transfer can be developed for some situations. This, however, is not attempted in this text. The postulate of an effective film is explained by reference to Figure 3.2.

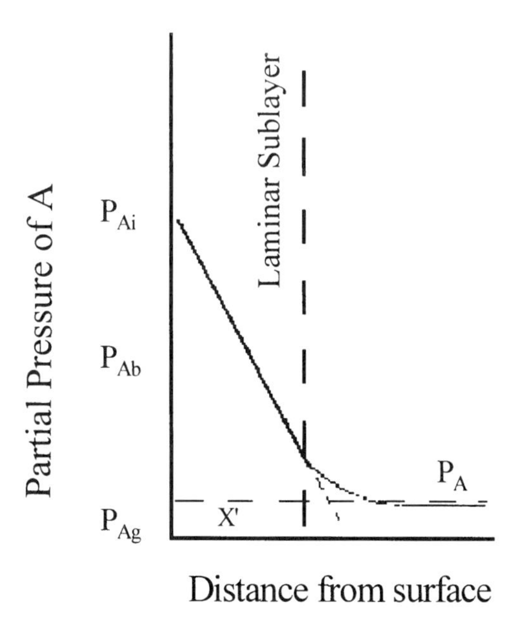


**FIGURE 3.2** Mass transfer at a boundary.

As gas flows over a surface and equimolecular counterdiffusion of components A and B occurs, component A moves away from the surface and component B moves toward the surface. The variation in partial pressure of A with distance from the surface is shown in Figure 3.2. At the surface the value is $P_{Ai}$. A linear fall to $P_{Ab}$ occurs over the laminar sublayer. Beyond this the partial pressure falls less steeply to the value $P_A$ at the edge of the boundary layer. A value slightly higher than this, $P_{Ag}$, is the average partial pressure of A in the entire system. In general, the gas content of the laminar layer is so small that $P_A$ and $P_{Ag}$ are virtually equal. If molecular diffusion were solely responsible for diffusion, $P_{Ag}$ would be reached at some fictitious distance, $x'$, from the surface, over which the concentration gradient $(P_{Ai} - P_{Ag})/x'$ exists. The molar rate of mass transfer would then be

$$N_A = \frac{D}{RT} \frac{P_{Ai} - P_{Ag}}{x'}$$

However, $x'$ is not known and this equation may be written

$$N_A = \frac{k_g}{RT}(P_{Ai} - P_{Ag}) \tag{3.5}$$

where $k_g$ is a mass transfer coefficient, the units of which are m s$^{-1}$. Since $C_A = P_A/RT$, we can also write

$$N_A = k_g(C_{Ai} - C_{Ag})$$

where $C_{Ai}$ and $C_{Ag}$ are the gas concentrations at either side of the film. Similar equations describe the diffusion of B in the opposite direction.

Diffusion across a liquid film is described by

$$N_A = k_l(C_{Ai} - C_{Al}) \tag{3.6}$$

where $C_{Ai}$ is the concentration of component A at the interface and $C_{Al}$ is its concentration in the bulk of the phase.

In all cases the mass transfer coefficient depends on the diffusivity of the transferred material and the thickness of the effective film. The latter is largely determined by the Reynolds number of the moving fluid—that is, its average velocity, its density, its viscosity, and some linear dimension of the system. Dimensional analysis gives the relation

$$\frac{kd}{D} = \text{constant } (\text{Re})^q \left(\frac{\eta}{\rho D}\right)$$

where Re is the Reynolds number, $k$ is the mass transfer coefficient, $D$ is the diffusivity, and $d$ is a dimension characterizing the geometry of the system.

This relation is analogous to the expression for heat transfer by forced convection given in Chapter 2. The dimensionless group $kd/D$ corresponds to the Nusselt group in heat transfer. The parameter $\eta/\rho D$ is known as the Schmidt number, Sc, and is the mass transfer counterpart of the Prandtl number. For example, the evaporation of a thin liquid film at the wall of a pipe into a turbulent gas is described by the equation

$$\frac{kd}{D} = 0.023\ \mathrm{Re}^{0.8}\ \mathrm{Sc}^{0.33}$$

Although the equation expresses experimental data, comparison with equation 2.13 from the heat transfer section again demonstrates the fundamental relation of heat and mass transfer.

Similar relations have been developed empirically for other situations. The flow of gases normal to and parallel to liquid surfaces can be applied to drying processes, and the agitation of solids in liquids can provide information for crystallization or dissolution. The final correlation allows estimation of the mass transfer coefficient with reasonable accuracy.

## 3.6 INTERFACIAL MASS TRANSFER

So far, only diffusion in the boundary layers of a single phase has been discussed. In practice, however, two phases are normally present, and mass transfer across the interface must occur. On a macroscopic scale the interface can be regarded as a discrete boundary. On the molecular scale, however, the change from one phase to another takes place over several molecular diameters. Due to the movement of molecules, this region is in a state of violent change, the entire surface layer changing many times a second. Transfer of molecules at the actual interface is, therefore, virtually instantaneous, and the two phases are at this point in equilibrium.

Since the interface offers no resistance, mass transfer between phases can be regarded as the transfer of a component from one bulk phase to another through two films in contact, each characterized by a mass transfer coefficient. This is the two-film theory and is the simplest of the theories of interfacial mass transfer. For the transfer of a component from a gas to a liquid, the theory is described in Figure 3.3. Across the gas film, the concentration, expressed as partial pressure, falls from a bulk concentration $P_{\mathrm{Ag}}$ to an interfacial concentra-

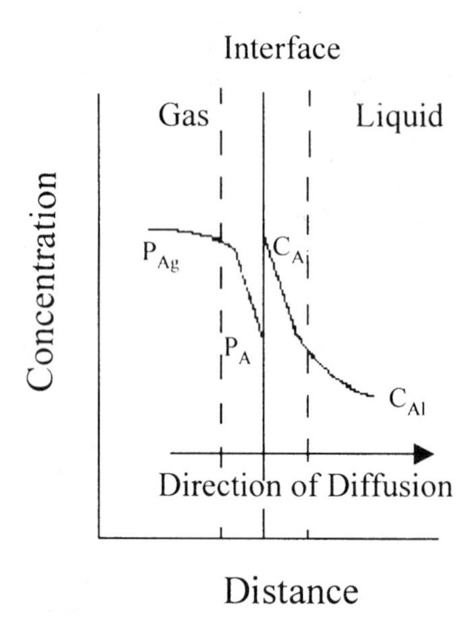


**FIGURE 3.3** Interfacial mass transfer.

tion $P_{Ai}$. In the liquid the concentration falls from an interfacial value $C_{Ai}$ to a bulk value $C_{Al}$.

At the interface equilibrium conditions exist. The break in the curve is due to the different affinity of component A for the two phases and the different units expressing concentration. The bulk phases are not, of course, at equilibrium, and it is the degree of displacement from equilibrium conditions that provides the driving force for mass transfer. If these conditions are known, an overall mass transfer coefficient can be calculated and used to estimate the rate of mass transfer.

Transfer of a component from one mixed phase to another, as described previously, occurs in several processes. Liquid-liquid extraction, leaching, gas adsorption, and distillation are examples. In other processes, such as drying, crystallization, and dissolution, one phase may consist of only one component. Concentration gradients are set up in one phase only with the concentration at the interface given by the relevant equilibrium conditions. In drying, for example, a layer of air in equilibrium, (i.e., saturated with the liquid) is postulated at the liquid surface, and mass transfer to a turbulent airstream is described by equation 3.5. The interfacial partial pressure is the vapor pressure of the liquid at the temperature of the surface. Similarly, dissolution is described by equation 3.6, the interfacial concentration being the saturation concentration. The rate of solution is determined by the difference between this concentration, the concentration in the bulk solution, and the mass transfer coefficient.

# 4

# Powders

Powders are employed in many pharmaceutical processes. They are more difficult to handle and process than liquids and gases primarily because their flow properties are fundamentally different. Unlike fluids, a particulate mass will resist stresses less than a limiting value without continuous deformation, and many common powders will not flow because the stresses imposed, for example, by gravity are insufficiently high. Often additional processes that improve flow, such as granulation and fluidization, are adopted to facilitate powder transport and powder feeding.

Another important property of powders is the manner in which the particles of a powder pack together to form a bed and its influence on bulk density. The latter is the ratio of the mass of the powder to its total volume, including voids. Unlike fluids, it varies greatly with the particle size, distribution, and shape of the particles because they affect the closeness of packing and the fraction of the bed that is void. Vibration and tapping, which cause rearrangement of the particles and a decrease in the void fraction, increase the bulk density. In several processes, these factors are important because the powder is subdivided and measured by volume. Variation of bulk density then causes variation in weight and dose. The variation in the weight of compressed tablets is an excellent example of this effect. The manner of packing also influences the behavior of a bed when it is compressed.

Finally, in a static condition, there is no leveling at the free surface of a bed of powder, nor is pressure transmitted downward through the bed. Instead, the walls of the containing vessel carry the weight of the bed.

## 4.1 PARTICLE PROPERTIES

### 4.1.1 Origins

In order to understand particle properties it is important to consider their origins. Particles may be produced by different processes that can be regarded as constructive or destructive (Hickey, 1993). Constructive methods include crystallization, precipitation, and condensation. Destructive methods include milling and spray-drying.

The most common methods of bulk manufacture are crystallization or precipitation from saturated solutions. These solutions are saturated by exceeding the solubility limit in one of several ways (Martin, 1993). Adding excess solid in the form of nucleating crystals results in crystallization from saturated solution. This can be controlled by reducing the temperature of the solution, thereby reducing the solubility. For products that can be melted at relatively low temperatures, heating and cooling can be used to invoke a controlled crystallization. The addition of a cosolvent with different capacity to dissolve the solute may also be used to reduce the solubility and result in precipitation. In the extreme a chemical reaction or complexation occurs to produce a precipitate (e.g., amine-phosphate/sulfate interactions; Fung, 1990) crystallization. Condensation from vapors is a technical possibility and has been employed for aerosol products (Pillai et al., 1993) but has little potential as a bulk manufacturing process.

Milling (Carstensen, 1993) and spray-drying (Masters, 1991) may be described as destructive methods since they take bulk solid or liquid and increase the surface area by significant input of energy, thereby producing small discrete particles or droplets. The droplets produced by spraying may then be dried to produce particles of pure solute. A variety of mills are available distinguished by their capacity to introduce energy into the powder. Spray dryers are available which may be utilized to produce powders from aqueous or nonaqueous solutions (Sacchetti and Van Oort, 1996).

### 4.1.2 Structure

The structure of particles may be characterized in terms of crystal system and crystal habit. The crystal system can be defined by the lattice group spacing and bond angles in three dimensions. Consequently, in the simplest form a crystal may be described by the distance between planes of atoms or molecules in three dimensions ($a$, $b$, and $c$) and by the angles between these planes ($\alpha$, $\beta$, and $\gamma$), where each angle is opposite the equivalent dimension (e.g., $\alpha$ opposite $a$). These angles and distances are determined by X-ray diffraction utilizing Bragg's law (Mullin, 1993). Crystals may be considered as polygons wherein the numbers of faces, edges, and vertices are defined by Euler's law. There are more than 200 possible permutations of crystal system based on this definition. In practice, each of these geometries can be classified into seven specific categories of crystal system: cubic, monoclinic, triclinic, hexagonal, trigonal, orthorhombic, and tetragonal.

Once the molecular structure of crystals has been established, the manner in which crystal growth occurs from solution is dictated by inhibition in any of the three dimensions. Inhibition of growth occurs because of differences in surface free energy or surface energy density. These differences may be brought about by regions of different polarity at the surface, charge density at the surface, the orientation of charged side groups on the molecules, the location of solvent at the interface, or the adsorption of other solute molecules (e.g., surfactant). Crystal growth gives rise to particles of different crystal habit. It is important to recognize that different crystal habits, or superficial appearance, do not imply different lattice group spacing, as defined by the crystal system. Also it is possible that products may be produced by any of the methods described that have no regular structure or specific orientation of molecules, which are, by definition, amorphous.

### 4.1.3 Properties

Properties dictated by the method of manufacture include particle size and distribution, shape, specific surface area, true density, tensile strength, melting point, and polymorphic form. Arising from these fundamental physicochemical properties are other properties such as solubility and dissolution rate.

Polymorphism, or the ability of crystals to exhibit different crystal lattice spacings under different conditions (usually of temperature or moisture content), can be evaluated by thermal techniques. Differential scanning calorimetry may be used to determine the energy requirements for rearranging molecules in the lattice as they convert from one form to another. This difference between polymorphic forms of the same substance can also be detected by assessing their solubility characteristics.

## 4.2 PARTICLE INTERACTIONS

The attraction between particles or between particles and a containing boundary influences the flow and packing of powders. If two particles are placed together, the cohesive bond is normally very much weaker than the mechanical strength of the particles themselves. This may be due to the distortion of the crystal lattice, which prevents correct alignment of the atoms, or the adsorption of surface films. These prevent contact of the surfaces and usually, but not always, decrease cohesion. Low cohesion is also the result of small area of contact between the surfaces. On a molecular scale, surfaces are very rough, and the real area of contact is very much smaller than the apparent area. Finally, the structure of the surface may differ from the interior structure of the particle. Nevertheless, the cohesion and adhesion that occur with all particles are appreciable. They are normally ascribed to nonspecific van der Waals forces, although in moist materials a moisture layer can confer cohesiveness by the action of surface tension at the points of contact. For this reason, an increase in humidity can produce a sudden increase in cohesiveness and the complete loss of mobility in a powder that ceases to flow and pour. The acquisition of an electric charge by frictional movement between particles is another mechanism by which particles cohere together or adhere to containers.

These effects depend on the chemical and physical form of the powder. They normally oppose the gravitational and momentum forces acting on a particle during flow and therefore become more effective as the weight or size of the particle decreases. Cohesion and adhesion increase as the size decreases because the number of points in contact in a given area of apparent contact increases. The effects of cohesion often predominate at sizes less than 100 micrometers and powders will not pass through quite large orifices, and vertical walls of a limited height appear in a free surface. The magnitude of cohesion also increases as the bulk density of the powder increases.

Cohesion also depends on the time for which contact is made. This is not fully understood but may be due to the gradual squeezing of air and adsorbed gases from between the approaching surfaces. The result, however, is that a system which flows under certain conditions may cease to flow when these conditions are restored after interruption. This is of great importance in the storage and intermittent delivery of powders. Fluctuating humidity can also destroy flow properties if a water-soluble component is present in the powder. The alternating processes of dissolution and crystallization can produce very strong bonds between particles which cement the mass together.

### 4.2.1 Measurement of the Effects of Cohesion and Adhesion

Measuring the cohesion between two particles or the adhesion of a particle to a boundary is difficult, although several methods can be used. More commonly, these effects are assessed by studying an assembly of particles in the form of a bed or a heap. Flow and other properties of the powder are then predicted from these studies.

The most commonly observed and measured property of a heap is the maximum angle at which a free powder surface can be inclined to the horizontal. This is the angle of repose and it can be measured in a number of ways, four of which are shown in Figure 4.1. The angle depends to some extent on the method chosen and the size of the heap. Minimum angles are about 25°, and powders with repose angles of less than 40° flow well. If the angle is over 50°, the powder flows with difficulty or not at all.

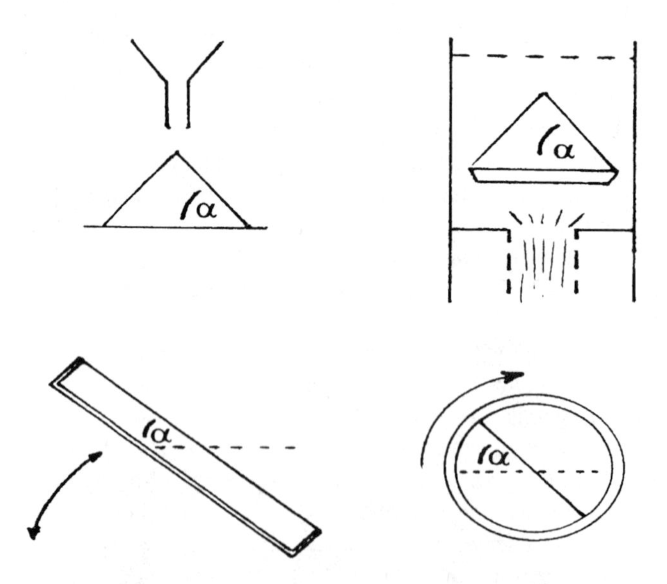


**FIGURE 4.1** Measurement of the angle of repose, $\alpha$.

The angle, which is related to the tensile strength of a powder bed, increases as the particle shape departs from sphericity and as the bulk density increases. Above 100 microns, it is independent of particle size, but below this value it increases sharply. The effect of humidity on cohesion and flow is reflected in the repose angle. Moist powders form an irregular heap with repose angles of up to 90°.

A more fundamental measure is the tensile stress necessary to divide a powder bed. The powder may be dredged onto a split plate or, in a more refined apparatus, contained within a split cylinder and carefully consolidated. The stress is found from the force required to break the bed and the area of the divided surface. The principles of this method are shown in Figure 4.2(a), and stresses of up to 100 $N/m^2$ are necessary to divide a bed of fine powders. Values increase as the bulk density increases. Changes in cohesiveness with time and the severe changes in the flow properties of some powders that occur when the relative humidity exceeds 80% can be assessed with this apparatus.

Apparatus for shearing a bed of powder is shown diagrammatically in Figure 4.2(b). The shear stress at failure is measured while the bed is constrained under a normal stress. The latter can be varied. The relation between these stresses, a subject fully explored in the science of soil mechanics, is used in the design of bins and hoppers for storage and delivery of powders.

The adhesion of particles to surfaces can be studied in a number of ways. Measuring the size of the particles retained on an upturned plate is a useful qualitative test. A common method measures the angle of inclination at which a powder bed slides on a surface, the bed itself remaining coherent.

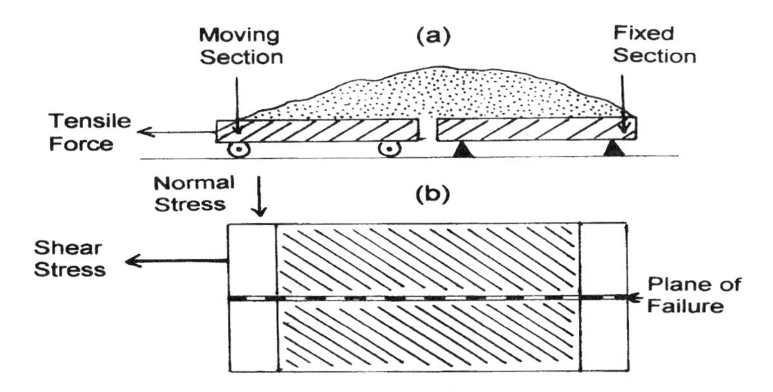


**FIGURE 4.2** Measuring the (a) tensile and (b) shear strength of a powder bed.

## 4.3 POWDER FLOW

The physics of powder flow has been studied thoroughly (Crowder and Hickey, 2000). However, it is only recently that this body of knowledge has been fully applied to pharmaceutical systems. Pharmaceutical applications exist for specific unit operations. The gravity flow of powders in chutes and hoppers and the movement of powders through a constriction occur in tabletting, encapsulation, and many processes in which a powder is subdivided for packing into final containers. In many cases, the accuracy of weight and dose depends on the regularity of flow. The flow of powders is extremely complex and is influenced by many factors. A profile in two dimensions of the flow of granular solids through an aperture is shown in Figure 4.3. Particles slide over A while A slides over B; B moves slowly over the stationary region E. Material is fed into zone C and moves downward and inward to a tongue D. Here, packing is less dense, particles move more quickly, and bridges and arches formed in the powder collapse. Unless the structure is completely emptied, powder in region E never flows through the aperture. If, in use, a container is partially emptied and partially filled, this material may spoil. If the container is narrow, region E *is* absent and the whole mass moves downward, the central part of region C occupying the entire tube.

For granular solids, the relation between mass flow rate, $G$, and the diameter of a circular orifice, $D_O$, is expressed by the equation

$$G = \text{Constant} \cdot D_O^a H^b$$

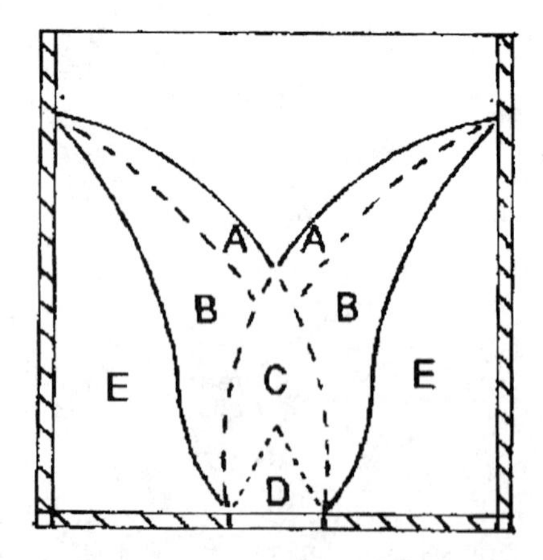


**FIGURE 4.3** Profile of granules flow through an orifice.

where $H$ is the height of the bed and $a$ and $b$ are constants. For a wide variety of powders, the constant $a$ lies between 2.5 and 3.0. If the height of the bed is several times that of the orifice, $H$ lies between 0 and 0.05. The absence of a pressure-depth relation, already observed in a static bed, seems, therefore, to persist in dynamic conditions.

The relation between mass flow rate and particle size is more complex. With an orifice of given size and shape, the flow increases as the particle size decreases until a maximum rate is reached. With further decrease in size and increase in cohesiveness, flow decreases and becomes irregular. Arches and bridges form above the aperture and flow stops. Determining the minimum aperture through which a powder will flow without assistance is a useful laboratory exercise. The distribution of particle sizes also affects the flow in a given system. Often, the removal of the finest fraction greatly improves flow. On the other hand, the addition of very small quantities of fine powder can, in some circumstances, improve flow. This is probably due to adsorption of these particles onto the original material, preventing close approach and the development of strong cohesional bonds. Magnesia and talc, for example, promote the flow of many cohesive powders. These materials, which can be called *glidants*, are useful additives when good flow properties of a powder are required.

Vibration and tapping may maintain or improve the flow of cohesive powders by preventing or destroying the bridges and arches responsible for irregular movement or blockage. Vibration and tapping to initiate flow are less satisfactory because the associated increase in bulk density due to closer packing renders the powder more cohesive.

## 4.4 PACKING OF POWDERS

Bulk density, already defined, and porosity are terms used to describe the degree of consolidation in a powder. The porosity, $\varepsilon$, is the fraction of the total volume which is void, often expressed as a percentage. It is related to the bulk density, $\rho_b$, by the equation

$$\varepsilon = 1 \frac{\rho_b}{\rho} \tag{4.1}$$

where $\rho$ is the true density of the powder.

When spheres of equal size are packed in a regular manner, the porosity can vary from a maximum of 46% for a cubical arrangement to a minimum of 26% for a rhombohedral array. These extremes are shown in Figure 4.4.

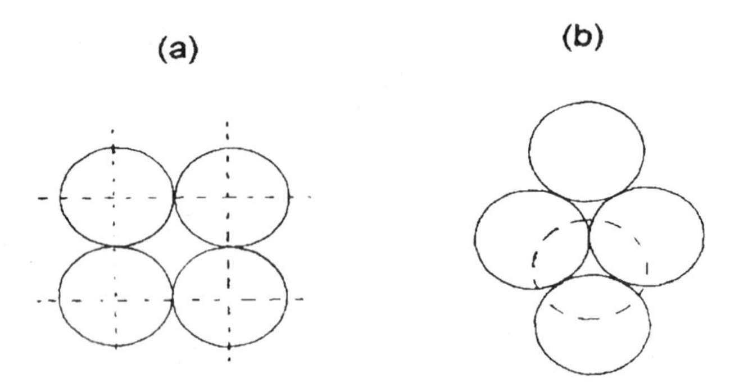


**FIGURE 4.4** Systematic packing of spheres.

For ideal systems of this type, the porosity is independent of particle size. In practice, of course, packing is not regular. Cubic packing, obtained when the next layer is placed directly on top of the four spheres above, is the most open packing, as shown in Figure 4.4(a). Rhombohedral packing, obtained when the next layer is built around the sphere shown in a broken line in Figure 4.4(b), is the closest packing.

Nevertheless, for coarse, isodiametric particles with a narrow range of sizes, the porosity is remarkably constant at between 37% and 40%. Lead shot, for example, packs with the same porosity as a closely graded sand. With wider size distributions, the porosity decreases because some packing of fine particles in the interstices between the coarsest particles becomes possible. These effects are absent in fine powders. Due to their more cohesive nature, the porosity increases as the particles become finer and variation in the size distribution has little effect.

In any irregular array, the porosity increases as particle shape departs from sphericity because open packing and bridging become more common. A flaky material, such as crushed mica, packs with a porosity of about 90%. Roughness of the particles' surface increases porosity.

In operations in which powders are poured, chance packing occurs and porosity is subject to the operation's speed and degree of agitation. If the powder is poured slowly, each particle can find a stable position in the developing surface. Interstitial volumes are small, the number of contacts with neighboring particles is high, and the porosity is low. If pouring is quick, there is insufficient time for stable packing, bridges are created as particles fall together, and a bed of higher porosity is formed. Vibration opposes open packing and the formation of bridges. It is often deliberately applied when closely packed powder beds are required.

Packing at a boundary differs from packing in the bulk of a powder. The boundary normally creates a region of more open packing, several particle layers in extent. This is important when particles are packed into small volumes. If the particles are relatively large, the region of expanded packing and low bulk density will be extensive and, for these conditions, the weight of material that fills the volume will decrease as particle size increases. With finer powders the opposite is true, and cohesiveness causes the weight of powder which fills a volume to decrease as particle size decreases. There is, therefore, some size of particle for which the capacity of a small volume is a maximum. This depends on the dimensions of the space into which the particles are packed.

## 4.5 GRANULATION

*Granulation* is a term for several processes used to produce materials in the form of coarse particles. In pharmacy, it is closely associated with the preparation of compressed tablets. Discussion is here limited to a general account of the process.

Ideally, granulation yields coarse isodiametric particles with a very narrow size distribution. The several advantages of this form can be inferred from the foregoing discussion. Granules flow well. They feed evenly from chutes and hoppers and pack into small volumes without great variation of weight. Segregation in a mixture of powders is prevented if the mixture is granulated. Each granule contains the correct proportions of the components so that segregation of granules cannot cause inhomogeneity in the mixture. The hazards of dust are eliminated and granules are less susceptible to lumping and caking. Finally, granular materials fluidize well, and a material may be granulated to gain the advantages of this process.

The starting materials for granulation vary from fine powders to solutions. Methods can be classified as wet or dry granulation. In the latter, a very coarse material is comminuted and classified. If the basic material is a fine powder, it is first aggregated by pressure with punches and dies, to give tablets or briquettes, or by passage through rollers, to give a sheet that is then broken.

In wet methods a liquid binder is added to a fine powder. If the proportion added converts the powder to a crumbly adhesive mass, it can be granulated by forcing it through a screen with an impeller. The wet granules are then dried and classified. If a wetter mass is made, it can be granulated by extrusion. Alternatively, the powder can be rotated in a pan and granulating fluid added until agglomeration occurs. Granule growth depends critically on the amount of fluid added and other variables, such as the particle's size and pan speed and the surface tension of the granulating fluid, must be closely controlled.

Granular materials are also prepared by spray-drying and by crystallization.

## 4.6 FLUIDIZATION

The movement of fluids through a fixed bed was described in Chapter 1. If the fluid velocity is low, the same situation is found when fluid is driven upward through a loose particulate bed. At higher velocities, however, frictional drag causes the particles to move into a more expanded packing which offers less resistance to flow. At some critical velocity, the particles are just touching and the pressure drop across the bed just balances its weight. This is the point of incipient fluidization; beyond it true fluidization occurs, the bed acquiring the properties of surface leveling and flow.

If the fluid is a liquid, increase in velocity causes the quiescent bed to rock and break, allowing individual particles to move randomly in all directions. Increase in velocity causes progressive thinning of this system. In fluidization by gases, the behavior of the bed is quite different. Although much of the gas passes between individual particles in the manner already described, the remainder passes in the form of bubbles so that the bed looks like a boiling liquid. Bubbles rise through the bed, producing an extensive wake from which material is continually lost and gained, and breaking at the surface distributes powder widely. This mixing mechanism is effective, and any nonhomogeneity in the bed is quickly destroyed. Rates of heat and mass transfer in the bed are therefore high.

Bubble size and movement vary in different systems. In general, both decrease as particle size decreases. As the size decreases and the powder becomes more cohesive, fluidization becomes more difficult. Eventually, bubbles do not form and very fine powders cannot be fluidized in this way.

The final stage of fluidization occurs at very high velocities when, in liquid and gaseous systems, the particles become entrained in the fluid and are carried along with it. These conditions are used to convey particulate solids from one place to another.

## 4.7 MIXING AND BLENDING

Mixing and blending may be achieved by rotating or shearing the powder bed. Mixing two or more components that may differ in composition, particle size, or some other physicochemical property is brought about through a sequence of events. Most powders at rest occupy a small volume such that it would be difficult to force two static powder beds to mix. The first step in a mixing process, therefore, is to dilate the powder bed. This second step, which may be concurrent with the first, is to shear the powder bed. Ideally, shearing occurs at the level of planes of individual particles. The introduction of large interparticulate spaces is achieved by rotating the bed. A V blender or a barrel roller are classical examples of systems which, by rotating through 360°, dilate the powder bed while, through the influence of gravity, shearing planes of particles. A planetary mixer uses blades to mechanically dilate and shear the powder. Each of these systems is a batch process. A ribbon blender uses a screwing action to rotate and shear the bed from one location to another in a continuous process.

Since the shearing of particles in a bed to achieve a uniform mix or blend is a statistical process, it must be monitored for efficiency. Sample thieves are employed to probe the powder bed, with minimal disturbance, and draw samples for analysis. These samples are then analyzed for the relevant dimension for mixing, e.g., particle sizes, drug, or excipient content. Statistical mixing parameters have been derived based on the mean and standard deviation of samples taken from various locations in a blend at various times during the processing (Carstensen, 1993). In large-scale mixers random number tables may be employed to dictate sample sites. There is a considerable science of sampling that can be brought to bear on this problem (Thompson, 1992). The sample size for pharmaceutical products is ideally of the scale of the unit dose. This is relevant as it relates to the likely variability in the dose that in turn relates to the therapeutic effect. In the case of small unit doses the goal should be to sample at a size within the resolution of the sample thief.

## 4.8 CONCLUSION

The origins, structure, and properties of particles within a powder dictate their dynamic performance. Gathering information on the physicochemical properties of powders is a prerequisite for interpreting and manipulating their flow and mixing properties. Flow properties are important to many unit processes in pharmacy, including transport and movement through hoppers, along conveyor belts, in granulators, and in mixers. Ultimately, the packing and flow properties can be directly correlated with the performance of the unit dose. Filling of capsules, blisters, or tablet dies, compression of tablets, and dispersion of powder aerosols all relate to powder properties.

# 5

# Air Conditioning and Humidification

Air conditioning for comfort means the provision of warm, filtered air. High moisture content or humidity is oppressive, but a low humidity may cause irritation by excessive loss of moisture from the skin. In some climates steps may be taken to add or remove water vapor from the air. The air is cleaned, usually by passage through a fabric filter which may be dry or moistened with a viscous liquid, and heated electrically or by banks of finned tubes supplied with steam or hot water over which the air is blown. Electrostatic precipitation provides an alternative method of air cleaning. The fine particles entrained in the air are charged by the absorption of electrons as they pass between two electrodes. The charged particle then migrates in the electrical field and is finally arrested on one electrode.

The same general principles apply to the supply of air in some pharmaceutical processes. However, the control of its quality may be more stringent. In areas in which sterile materials are made and handled, for example, the air cleaning must remove bacteria. In other processes, it may be necessary to remove water vapor. The flow of powders is a sensitive function of moisture content. The equilibrium moisture content of a material is determined by the humidity. Some tableting processes break down if the humidity is too high. In such processes, the scale of the air conditioning varies. It may be necessary to supply a whole room with air of a certain quality. Alternatively, conditioning may be restricted to a small area surrounding a particular piece of equipment.

## 5.1 VAPOR AND GAS MIXTURES

The humidity of a vapor-gas mixture is defined as the mass of vapor associated with unit mass of the gas. This principle is generally applicable to any vapor present in any noncondensable gas. In this section, however, only water vapor in air is considered. The percent humidity is the ratio of ambient humidity to the humidity of the saturated gas at the same temperature, expressed as a percentage. These terms should be carefully distinguished from the relative humidity with which they are distantly related. The relative humidity is the ratio of the partial pressure of the vapor in the gas to the partial pressure when the gas is saturated. This is also usually expressed as a percentage. The relative humidity of a given vapor-gas mixture changes with temperature, but the humidity does not.

The study of the properties of the air-water vapor mixture is called psychrometry, and data is presented in the form of psychrometric charts. These take various forms and present various data (Perry and Chilton, 1973). In

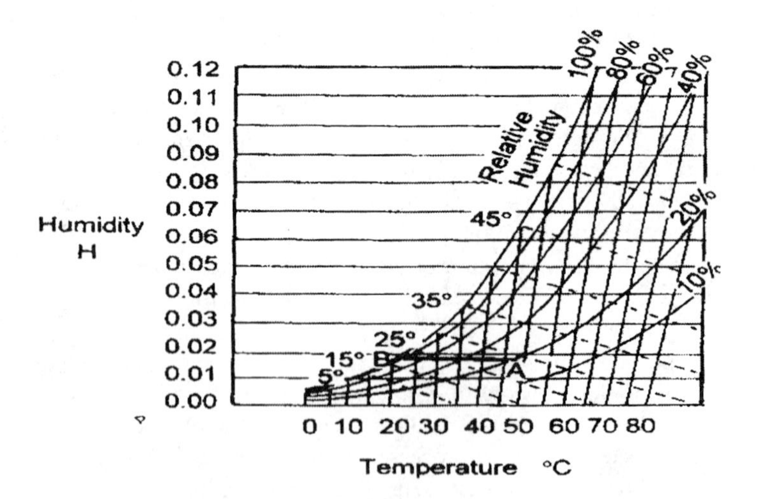


**FIGURE 5.1** A psychrometric chart that can be used to determine the humidity, dew point, and wet and dry bulb temperatures.

Figure 5.1, humidity is plotted as the ordinate and temperature as the abscissa. Percent relative humidity is then plotted as a series of curves running across the chart. The use of this simplified chart is demonstrated later in this chapter and the next.

## 5.2 HYGROMETRY, THE MEASUREMENT OF HUMIDITY

The accurate determination of the air's humidity is carried out gravimetrically. The water vapor present in a known volume of air is chemically absorbed with a suitable reagent and weighed. In other less laborious methods, the humidity is derived from the dew point or the wet bulb depression of a water vapor-air mixture.

The dew point is the temperature at which a vapor-gas mixture becomes saturated when cooled at constant pressure. If air of the condition denoted by point A in Figure 5.1 is cooled, the relative humidity increases until the mixture is fully saturated. This condition is given by point B where the temperature coordinate is the dew point. This can be measured rapidly by evaporating ether in a silvered bulb. The temperature at which dew deposits from the surrounding air is noted, and the humidity is read directly from a psychrometric chart.

Humidity derivation from the wet bulb depression requires a preliminary study of the transfer of mass and heat at a boundary between air and water. Since this process is also important in the study of drying, a detailed explanation is set out. If a small quantity of water evaporates into a large volume of air, conditions which make the change in humidity negligible, the latent heat of evaporation is supplied from the sensible heat of the water. The latter cools and the temperature gradient between water and air promotes the flow of heat from the surrounding air to the surface. As the temperature falls, the rate of heat flow increases until it equals the rate at which heat is required for evaporation. The temperature at the surface then remains constant at what is known as the wet bulb temperature. The difference between the air temperature and the wet bulb temperature is the wet bulb depression. If these temperatures are denoted by $T_a$ and $T_{wb}$, the rate of heat transfer, $Q$, is

$$Q = hA(T_a - T_{wb}) \tag{5.1}$$

where $A$ is the area over which heat is transferred and $h$ is the heat transfer coefficient. Mass transfer of water vapor from the water surface to the air is described by the equation

$$N = \frac{k_g}{RT}(P_{wi} - P_{wa}) \tag{5.2}$$

where $P_{wi}$ is the partial pressure of water vapor at the surface, $P_{wa}$ is the partial pressure of water vapor in the air, $k_g$ is a mass transfer coefficient, and $N$ is the number of moles transferred from unit area in unit time. Rewriting this equation in terms of the mass, $W$, transferred at the whole surface in unit time, where $M_w$ is the molecular weight of water vapor, we get

$$W = \frac{M_w A}{RT} k_g(P_{wi} - P_{wa}) \tag{5.3}$$

where $A$ is the area of the surface. If the partial pressure of water vapor in a system has the value $P_w$, then, from the general gas equation, the mass of vapor in unit volume is $(P_w/RT)\ M_w$. Similarly, if the total pressure is $P$, the mass of air in unit volume is $[(P - P_w)/RT]/M_a$, where $M_a$ is the ''molecular weight'' of the air. The humidity, $H$, is the ratio of these two quantities:

$$H = \left(\frac{P_w}{P - P_w}\right)\frac{M_w}{M_a} \tag{5.4}$$

If $P \ggg P_w$, $H = (P_w/P)(M_w/M_a)$. Rearranging and substituting humidity for partial pressure in equation 5.3 give

$$W = \frac{PM_a}{RT} k_g A(H_i - H_a) \tag{5.5}$$

where $H_a$ is the humidity of the air and $H_i$ is the humidity at the surface. The latter is known from the vapor pressure of water at the wet bulb temperature. Since $PM_a/RT = \rho$, equation 5.5 can be written

$$W = \rho k_g A(H_i - H_a) \tag{5.6}$$

where $\rho$ is the density of the air. If the latent heat of evaporation is $\lambda$, the heat transfer rate necessary to promote this evaporation is

$$Q = \rho k_g A(H_i - H_a) \tag{5.7}$$

Equating expressions 2.7 and 5.7 then gives

$$H_i - H_a = \frac{h}{\rho k_g \lambda}(T_a - T_{wb}) \tag{5.8}$$

Both the heat and mass transfer coefficients are functions of air velocity. However, at air speeds greater than about 4.5 m $s^{-1}$, the ratio $h/k_g$ is approximately constant. The wet bulb depression is directly proportional to the difference between the humidity at the surface and the humidity in the bulk of the air.

In the wet and dry bulb hygrometers, the wet bulb depression is measured by two thermometers, one of which is fitted with a fabric sleeve wetted with water. These are mounted side by side and shielded from radiation, an effect neglected in the preceding derivation. Air is then drawn over the thermometers by a small fan. The derivation of the humidity from the wet bulb depression and a psychrometric chart will be discussed later.

Many wet and dry bulb hygrometers operate without any form of induced air velocity at the wet bulb. This may be explained by examining another air-water system. If a limited quantity of air and water is allowed to equilibrate in conditions in which heat is neither gained nor lost by the system, the air becomes saturated and the latent heat required for evaporation is drawn from both fluids, which will cool to the same temperature. This temperature is the adiabatic saturation temperature, $T_s$. It is a peculiarity of the air-water system that the adiabatic saturation temperature and the wet bulb temperature are the same. If water at this temperature is recycled in a system through which air is passing, the incoming air is cooled until it reaches the adiabatic saturation temperature, at which point it is saturated. The temperature of the water, on the other hand, remains constant, and all the latent heat required for evaporation is drawn from the sensible heat of the air. Equilibrium is then expressed by the following equation:

$$(T_a - T_\infty)S = (H_\infty - H_a)\lambda \tag{5.9}$$

where $T_a$ is the temperature of the incoming air, $S$ is its specific heat, $H_a$ and $H_\infty$ are the humidities of the incoming air and the saturated air, and $\lambda$ is the latent heat of evaporation for water.

The process of adiabatic saturation in which the humidity progressively rises and the temperature progressively falls is described on a humidity chart by adiabatic cooling lines which run diagonally to the saturation curve. Charts are specially constructed so that these lines become parallel.

If a wet and dry bulb hygrometer is exposed to still air, the region adjacent to the wet bulb closely resembles the system described. After a considerable period, equilibrium is attained and the wet bulb records the adiabatic saturation temperature.

When both wet and dry bulb temperatures have been found, the humidity is read from the psychrometric chart in the following way. The point on the saturation curve corresponding to the wet bulb temperature is first found. An adiabatic cooling line is then interpolated and followed until the coordinate corresponding to the dry bulb temperature is reached. The humidity is read from the other axis.

The change in the physical properties of a hair or fiber with change in humidity is utilized in many instruments. After calibration, they are suitable for use over a limited range of humidity.

## 5.3 HUMIDIFICATION AND DEHUMIDIFICATION

Most commonly, air is humidified by passage through a spray of water. Three methods are illustrated by the humidity diagrams in Figure 5.2. In the first, air at temperature $T_1$ is heated to $T_2$. The latter temperature is chosen so that adiabatic cooling and saturation followed by heating to $T_4$ will give a humidity rise from $H_1$ to $H_2$. The humidification stage is performed by passing the air

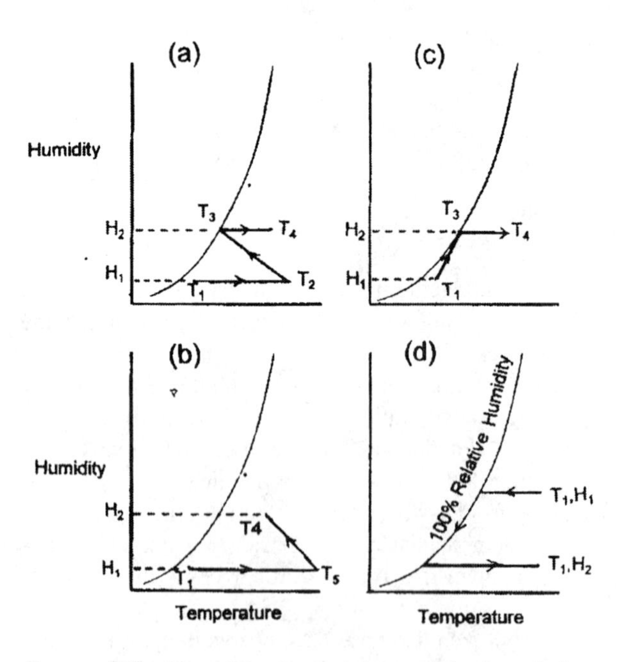


FIGURE 5.2 Humidification and dehumidification of air.

through water sprays at the adiabatic saturation temperature, $T_3$. Alternatively, the incoming air could be heated to $T_5$, air of the correct humidity emerging when it is adiabatically cooled to $T_4$ with water. In neither of these methods is control of the water temperature necessary. In the third method, air of humidity $H_1$ and temperature $T_1$ is passed through and saturated by a water spray maintained at $T_3$. On leaving the chamber, it is heated to $T_4$.

For small quantities of air, dehumidification is most easily accomplished by adsorbing water vapor with alumina or silica gel arranged in columns. These columns are mounted in pairs so that one can be regenerated while the other is in use. Alternatively, the air can be cooled below the dew point. Excess water vapor condenses and the cold saturated air is then reheated. For well-mixed gases, the process is described in Figure 5.2.

# 6

# Drying

Drying may be defined as the vaporization and removal of water or other liquid from a solution, suspension, or other solid-liquid mixture to form a dry solid. The change of phase from liquid to vapor distinguishes drying from mechanical methods of separating solids from liquids, such as filtration. The latter often precede drying since, where applicable, they offer a cost-effective method for removing a large part of the liquid.

Drying might still be confused with evaporation. Greater precision is not possible because the division of the two operations is to some extent arbitrary. Drying is normally associated with the removal of relatively small quantities of liquid to give a dry product. Evaporation is more often applied to the concentration of solutions. However exceptions to these generalizations occur.

Adjustment and control of moisture levels by drying are important in the manufacture and development of pharmaceutical products. Apart from the obvious requirement of dry solids for many operations, drying may be carried out to

1. Improve handling characteristics, as in bulk powder filling and other operations involving powder flow

2. Stabilize moisture-sensitive materials, such as aspirin and ascorbic acid

A wide range of drying equipment is available to meet these ends, but in practice the choice is limited by the scale of the operation and may be determined partly or completely by the thermal stability of the material and the physical form in which it is required. In the pharmaceutical industry, batch sizes are frequently small and of high value and the same dryer may be used to dry different materials. These factors limit the application of continuous dryers and promote the use of batch dryers that give low product retention and are easily cleaned. Recovery of solvents, where economically justified, may be another factor affecting choice of equipment.

## 6.1 THEORY OF DRYING

Theories of drying are limited in application in that drying times are normally experimentally determined. Nevertheless, an appreciation of the scope and limitations of the different drying methods is given. The following terms are employed in discussing drying: humidity, humidity of saturated air, relative humidity, wet bulb temperature, and adiabatic cooling line (see Chapter 5). Other terms may be defined as follows:

*Moisture content.* This is usually expressed as a weight per unit weight of dry solids.

*Equilibrium moisture content.* If a material is exposed to air at a given temperature and humidity, it will gain or lose moisture until equilibrium is reached. The moisture present at this point is defined as the equilibrium moisture content for the given exposure conditions. At a given temperature it varies with the partial pressure of the water vapor in the surrounding atmosphere. This is shown for a hypothetical hygroscopic material in Figure 6.1 in which the equilibrium moisture content is plotted against the relative humidity. Any moisture present in excess of the equilibrium moisture content is called *free water.*

Equilibrium moisture content curves vary greatly with the type of material examined. Insoluble, nonporous materials, such as talc or zinc oxide, give equilibrium moisture contents of almost zero over a wide humidity range. A moisture content of between 10% and 15% may be expected for cotton fabrics under normal atmospheric conditions. Drying below the equilibrium moisture content for room conditions may be deliberately undertaken, particularly if

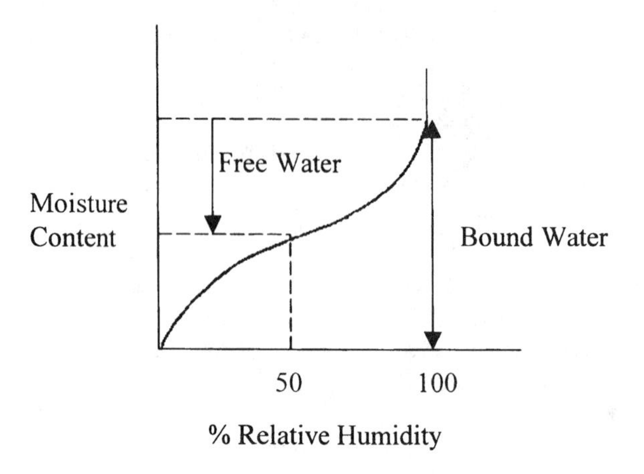


**FIGURE 6.1** Relation between equilibrium moisture content and relative humidity for a hygroscopic solid.

the material is unstable in the presence of moisture. Subsequent storage conditions then become important for product stability.

The equilibrium moisture content at 100% relative humidity represents the minimum amount of water associated with the solid that still exerts a vapor pressure equal to a separate water surface. If the humidity is reduced, only part of the water evaporates before a new equilibrium is established. The water retained at less than 100% relative humidity must, therefore, exert a vapor pressure below that of a dissociated water surface. Such water is called *bound water*. Unlike the equilibrium moisture content, bound water is a function of the solid only and not of the surroundings. Such water is usually held in small pores bound with highly curved menisci, is present as a solution, or is adsorbed on the surface of the solid.

The value of equilibrium moisture content curves is illustrated in Figure 6.2. The equilibrium moisture content of the antacid granules, composed of magnesium trisilicate granulated with syrup, is a sensitive function of relative humidity. If it is to be dried to a moisture content of 3%, air at a relative humidity of less than 35% must be used. With knowledge of the humidity of the circulating air, psychrometric charts may be used to determine the minimum air temperature that will dry the material to the required standard. (In fact, the temperature has an effect on the equilibrium moisture content that is independent of the humidity, but this can be neglected to a first approximation.) The lactose granulation, on the other hand, has a low sensitivity to rela-

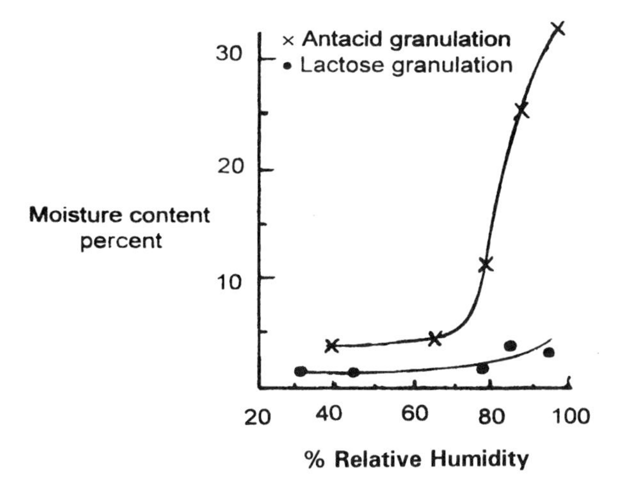


**Figure 6.2** Equilibrium moisture content curves for two tablet granulations.

tive humidity. Drying at low relative humidities derived from high air temperatures causes only a marginal decrease in the final moisture content, and the stability of the active ingredients associated with the lactose filler could be impaired. This argument may only be applied to the final moisture content. It is not related to the rate of drying, which would, of course, be greater at higher temperatures and lower humidities.

The effects of storage after drying may also be assessed from the equilibrium moisture content curves. Storage conditions are not critical for lactose granulation. If the antacid formulation was stored at a relative humidity of only 65% it would, given sufficient time, absorb moisture until the content was 9%. This could be associated with poor flow characteristics and its attendant difficulties during compression.

Dynamic vapor sorption techniques now exist which allow thorough studies of moisture association with solids under a wide range of relative humidity conditions based on microbalance technology.

## 6.2 EVAPORATION OF WATER INTO AN AIRSTREAM

The evaporation of moisture into a warm airstream, the latter providing the latent heat of evaporation, is a common drying mechanism although it is not easily adapted to the recovery of the liquid. We will first consider evaporation from a liquid surface which, with the passage of air, falls to the wet bulb temperature corresponding to the temperature and humidity of the air, as described in Chapter 5. The rate at which water vapor is transferred from the saturated layer at the surface to the drying stream is described by equation 3.5:

$$N = \frac{k_g}{RT} (P_{wi} - P_{wa}) \tag{3.5}$$

where $P_{wi}$ is the partial pressure of the water vapor at the surface, $P_{wa}$ is the partial pressure of water vapor in the air, $k_g$ is a mass transfer coefficient, and $N$ is the number of moles of vapor transferred from unit area in unit time. Rewriting this in terms of the total mass, $W$, transferred in unit time from the entire drying surface of area $A$; we obtain

$$W = \frac{M_w A}{RT} k_g (P_{wi} - P_{wa}) \tag{6.1}$$

where $M_w$ is the molecular weight of water vapor, $R$ is the gas constant, and $T$ is the absolute temperature.

The mass transfer coefficient, $k_g$, is a function of the temperature and the air's velocity and angle of incidence. A high velocity or angle of incidence diminishes the thickness of the stationary air layer in contact with the liquid surface and, therefore, lowers the diffusional resistance.

The rate of evaporation may also be expressed in terms of the heat transferred across the laminar film from the drying gases to the surface. This is described by equation 2.7:

$$Q = hA(T_a - T_s) \tag{2.7}$$

where $Q$ is the rate of heat transfer, $A$ is the area of the surface, $T_a$ and $T_s$ are the temperatures of the drying air and the surface, respectively, and $h$ is the heat transfer coefficient. The latter is also a function of air velocity and angle of impingement. If the latent heat of evaporation is $\lambda$, this affords a mass transfer rate, $W$, given by

$$W = \frac{hA}{\lambda} (T_a - T_s) \tag{6.2}$$

Equilibrium drying conditions are represented by the equality of relations 6.1 and 6.2. When these conditions pertain to drying, the surface temperature, $T_s$, which is the wet bulb temperature, is normally much lower than the temperature of the drying gases. This is of great importance in the drying of thermolabile materials.

If solids are present in the surface, the rate of evaporation is modified, the overall effect depending on the structure of the solids and the moisture content.

## 6.3 STATIC BEDS OF NONPOROUS SOLIDS

Drying wet granular beds, the particles of which are not porous and are insoluble in the wetting liquid, has been extensively studied. The operation is presented as the relation of moisture content and drying time [Figure 6.3(a)]. Note that the equilibrium moisture content is approached slowly. A protracted period may be required for the removal of water just above the equilibrium value. This time is not justified if a small amount of water can be tolerated in further processing, and such a process indicates the importance of establishing realistic drying requirements. The stability of the solids, maintained, as shown later, at a temperature close to that of the drying air, may allow unnecessary deterioration.

The data has been converted to a curve relating the rate of drying to moisture content [Figure 6.3(b)]. The initial heating-up period during which equilibrium is established is short and has been omitted from both figures.

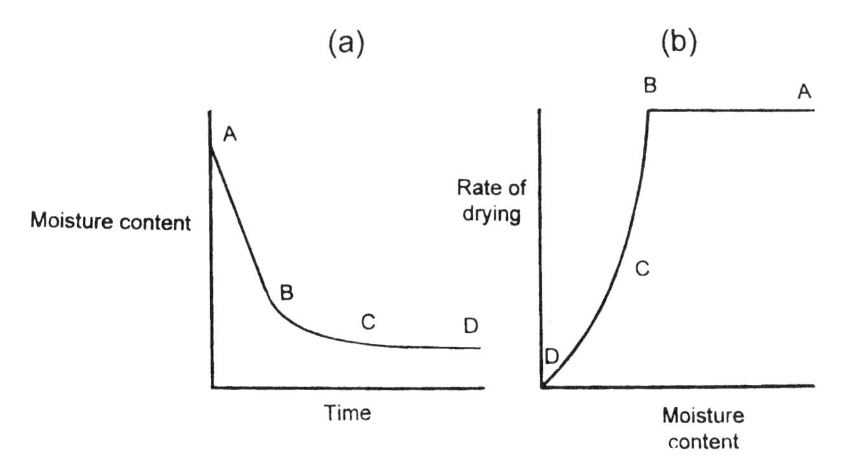


**FIGURE 6.3** (a) Moisture content vs. time of drying; (b) rate of drying vs. moisture content.

Assuming that sufficient moisture is initially present, the drying rate curve exhibits three distinct sections limited by points A, B, C, and D. In section A-B, called the *constant rate period*, it is considered that moisture is evaporating from a saturated surface at a rate governed by diffusion from the surface through the stationary air film in contact with it. An analogy with evaporation from a plain water surface can therefore be drawn. The drying rate during this period depends on the air temperature, humidity, and speed, which, in turn, determine the temperature of the saturated surface. Assuming that these are constant, all variables in the drying equations are fixed, and a constant rate of drying is established which is largely independent of the material being dried. The drying rate is somewhat lower than for a free-water surface and depends to some extent on the particle size of the solids. During the constant rate period, liquid must be transported to the surface at a rate sufficient to maintain saturation. The mechanism of transport is discussed later.

At the end of the constant rate period, B, a break in the drying curve occurs. This point is called the *critical moisture content*, and a linear fall in the drying rate occurs with further drying. This section, B-C, *is* called *the first falling rate period.* At and below the critical moisture content, the movement of moisture from the interior is no longer sufficient to saturate the surface. As drying proceeds, moisture reaches the surface at a decreasing rate, and the mechanism that controls its transfer will influence the rate of drying. Since the surface is no longer saturated, it tends to rise above the wet bulb temperature.

For any material, the critical moisture content decreases as the particle size decreases. Eventually, moisture does not reach the surface that becomes dry. The plane of evaporation recedes into the solid, the vapor reaching the surface by diffusion through the pores of the bed. This section is called the *second falling rate period* and is controlled by vapor diffusion, a factor largely independent of the conditions outside the bed but markedly affected by the particle size due to the latter's influence on the dimensions of pores and channels. During this period, the surface temperature approaches the temperature of the drying air.

Considerable migration of liquid occurs during the constant rate and first falling rate periods. Associated with the liquid are any soluble constituents that will form a concentrating solution in the surface layers as drying proceeds. Deposition of these materials takes place when the surface dries. Considerable segregation of soluble elements in the cake can occur, therefore, during drying.

If the soluble matter forms a skin or gel on drying rather than a crystalline deposit, a different drying curve (Figure 6.4) is obtained. The constant rate period is followed by a continuous fall in the drying rate in which no differentiation of first and second falling rate periods can be made. During this

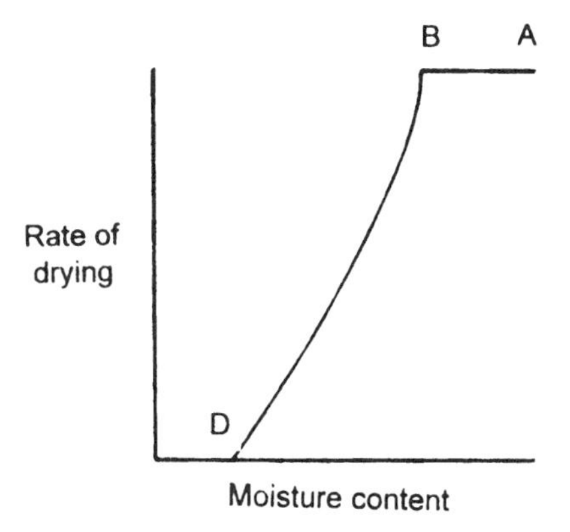


**FIGURE 6.4** Driving curve for a skin-forming material.

period, drying is controlled by diffusion through the skin that is continually increasing in thickness. Soap and gelatin are solutes that behave in this way.

## 6.4 THE INTERNAL MECHANISM OF DRYING

Extensive studies have been made to determine the nature of the forces that initially convey moisture to the surface at a rate sufficient to maintain saturation and their subsequent failure. Liquid movement may occur by diffusion under the concentration gradient created by water depletion at the surface by evaporation, as the result of capillary forces, through a cycle of vaporization and condensation, or by osmotic effects. Of these, capillary forces offer a coherent explanation for the drying periods of many materials.

If a tapered capillary is filled with water and exposed to a current of air, the meniscus at the smaller end remains stationary while the tube empties from the wider end. A similar situation exists in a wet particulate bed, and the phenomenon is explained by the concept of suction potential. A negative pressure exists below the meniscus of a curved liquid surface which is proportional to the surface tension, $\gamma$, and inversely proportional to the radius of curvature, $r$. (The meniscus is assumed to be part of a hemisphere.) This negative pressure or suction potential may be expressed as the height of liquid, $h$, it will support:

$$h = \frac{2\gamma}{\rho g r} \tag{6.3}$$

where $\rho$ is the density of the liquid. The suction potential, $h_x$, acting at a depth $x$ below the meniscus is then

$$h_x = h - x \tag{6.4}$$

The particles of the bed enclose spaces or pores connected by passages, the narrowest part of which is called the *waist*. The waist dimensions are determined by the size of the surrounding particles and the manner in which they are packed. In a randomly packed bed, pores and waists of varying sizes are found. Thus, the radius of a capillary running through the bed varies continuously. The depletion of water in this network is controlled by the waists because the radii of curvature are smaller and the suction potentials greater than for the pores. Depletion occurs in the following way. As evaporation proceeds, the water surface recedes into the waists of the top layer of particles and a suction potential develops. The maximum suction potential a waist can develop is called its "entry" suction potential and this potential is exceeded for larger waists by the suction potential developed by the smaller waists and transmitted through the continuous, connecting thread of liquid. The menisci in the larger waists then collapse and the pores they protect are emptied. A surface waist developing a suction potential, $h_s$, assuming an interconnecting thread of liquid, causes the collapse of an interior waist developing a suction potential, $h_i$, at a distance, $x$, below the surface if $h_s > h_i + x$. The liquid in the exposed pores is then lost at the surface by evaporation. This effect continues until a waist provides an opposing suction potential equal to or greater than the suction potential provided at that depth by the fine surface waist meniscus. The latter then collapses and the pore it protects is emptied.

By this mechanism, a meniscus in a fine surface waist holds its position and depletes the interior of moisture. If sufficient full surface waists are present, the constant rate period is maintained since the stationary air film in contact with the bed can be saturated. The first falling rate period indicates that insufficient full surface waists are present. Eventually, the collapse of all surface waists takes place, giving a breakdown of the capillary network supplying moisture to the surface, and the second falling rate period ensues.

## 6.5 STATIC BEDS OF POROUS SOLIDS

The drying curve obtained when the particles that compose the bed are themselves porous is shown in Figure 6.5. It differs from the curve obtained with nonporous materials in that the constant rate period is shorter. The rate of drying may be higher and is almost independent of particle size. The critical

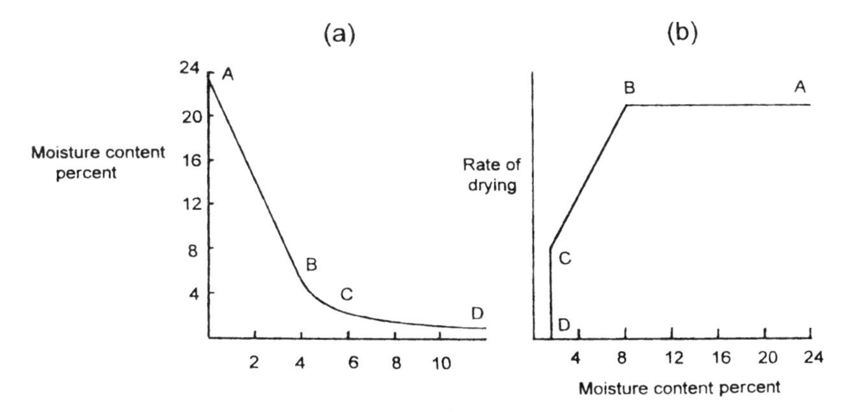


**FIGURE 6.5** Drying curves for a tablet granulation dried in a tray dryer.

moisture content is a function of the pore and particle sizes. During the first falling rate period, the rate of drying falls steeply due, it is thought, to the drying of the surface granules. The second falling rate period is influenced by the diffusion of moisture from within the particles.

## 6.6 THROUGH CIRCULATION DRYING

If the particles are in a suitable granular form, it is often possible to pass the airstream downward through the bed of solids. Drying will then follow the pattern described in previous sections except that each particle or agglomerate behaves as a drying bed. The surface area exposed to the drying gases is greatly increased, and drying rates 10 to 20 times greater than those encountered when air is passed over a free surface are obtained.

## 6.7 METHODS INVOLVING MOVEMENT OF THE SOLID

As an extension of drying by passing the airstream through a static bed of solids, it is possible to project air upward through the bed at a velocity high enough to fluidize the particles. Alternatively, the material may be mechanically subdivided and then introduced into the drying stream. Both methods give high drying rates due to high interfacial contact between the drying surfaces and the airstream. Fluidized bed dryers and spray dryers, respectively, use these principles.

## 6.8 OTHER METHODS OF DRYING

Apart from specialized dryers using infrared or dielectric heating, the chief method of passing heat into a drying solid, other than from a hot airstream, is by conduction from a heated surface. When a wet solid is placed in contact with a hot surface, subsequent events depend on the surface temperature relative to the liquid's boiling point, the nature of the solid, and the method of heating the surface. It is assumed here that the surface temperature is not hot enough for convective boiling to take place.

Consider first a cake of finely divided solids saturated with water. A temperature gradient will be established through the cake and evaporation from the free surface will take place at a rate governed entirely by the rate of heat input. During this period, the rate of evaporation and the temperature of a particular layer of cake are approximately constant. This continues until capillary forces are unable to transfer liquid to the free surface at the required rate. The temperature gradients during this period are given in Figures 6.6(a) and 6.6(b) for conditions in which the shelf temperature is below and above the boiling point of the liquid, respectively.

With a comparatively low heat flux, such that the partially dried cake can conduct heat away from the hot surface at the required rate, the free surface will dry and a fictitious drying line recedes slowly into the cake. The vapor diffuses through the dry cake to the free surface. The temperature gradient during this falling rate period is shown in Figure 6.6(c). If the heat flux is high, the point at which mobile water can no longer reach the surface is marked by the onset of drying in a layer adjacent to the hot surface, and vapor is forced through the wet cake above. As the solid dries, its temperature increases and a temperature gradient is established through the dry solids to the upward-receding drying line [Figure 6.6(d)]. The free surface of the solid appears wet and is at a constant temperature. These conditions are destroyed when the drying line reaches the surface.

In either case, a low and falling rate of drying will persist as the absorbed water is removed. In this form of drying, the heat treatment received by the solid is not uniform but depends on its position in the cake.

A hot surface may also be used to dry solutions, such as milk or plant extracts, which do not readily give porous, crystalline solids on concentration.

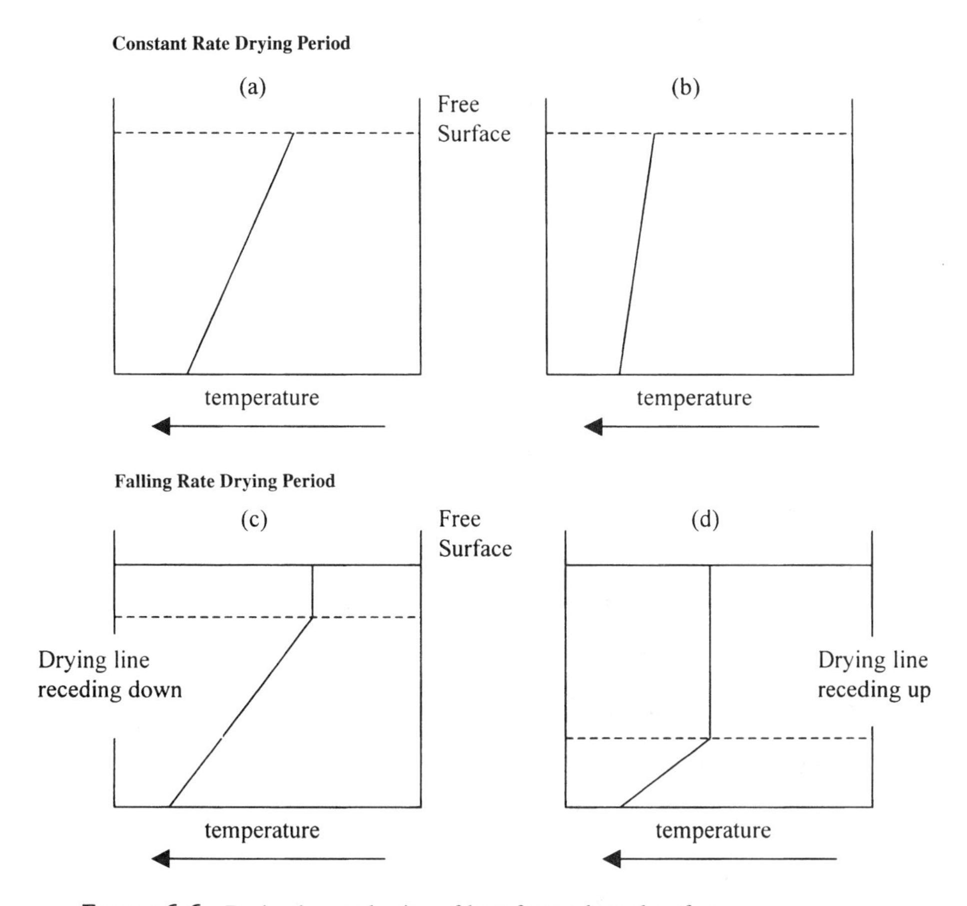


**FIGURE 6.6** Drying by conduction of heat from a heated surface

Apart from an initial constant rate period, when heat transfer is mainly convective, drying periods are ill-defined. As concentration proceeds, the liquor becomes more viscous and heat transfer is mainly by conduction. Large volume changes occur between initial and final stages. It is possible to dry thin films of solution to a solid film, but if deeper layers are taken a skin is frequently formed at the free surface that is almost impervious to the vapor. Frothing and drying to a porous, friable structure then occur. They may also occur if, during the upward recession of the drying line, the material above is too viscous to allow vapor to escape.

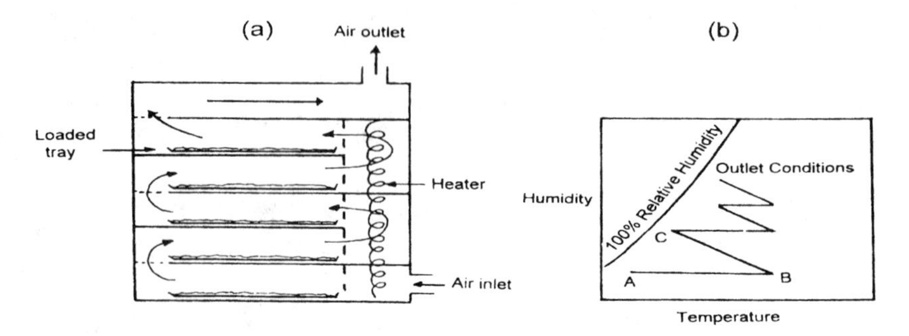


**FIGURE 6.7** (a) Tray dryer. (b) Temperature-humidity sequence of drying air.

## 6.9 SOLIDS MOVING OVER A HOT SURFACE

Conditions in which the solids move over a heated surface are employed in tumbling and agitated dryers. Drying rates are higher than those obtained in static beds because fresh solids are continually exposed to the hot surface. The heat treatment received by the solid will be more uniform.

## 6.10 BATCH DRYERS

### 6.10.1 Hot Air Ovens

Ovens operating by passing hot air over the surface of a wet solid that is spread over trays arranged in racks provide the simplest and cheapest dryer. On small installations, the air is passed over electrically heated elements and once through the oven. Larger units may employ steam-heated, finned tubes, and thermal efficiency is improved by recirculating the air. This is controlled by manually set dampers, and a common operating position gives 90% recirculation and 10% bleed-off. The heater bank is placed so that the solids do not receive radiant heat, and incoming air may be filtered. A typical hot air oven is illustrated schematically in cross section in Figure 6.7(a).

The temperature-humidity sequence of the circulating drying air is presented in Figure 6.7(b). The incoming air, at a temperature and humidity given by point A, is heated at constant humidity to point B and passed over the wet solid. The humidity rises and the temperature falls as the adiabatic cooling line is followed until the air leaves the tray in condition C. It is then recirculated to the heater; in Figure 6.7(b), two further cycles are shown.

We have assumed that all heat is drawn from the air and transmitted across the stationary air layer in contact with the drying surface, as described earlier. Surface temperatures are, in fact, modified by heat absorbed and conducted from unwetted surfaces, such as the underside of the tray, and by radiation.

The chief advantage of the hot air oven, apart from its low initial cost, is its versatility. With the exception of dusty solids, materials of almost any other physical form may be dried. Thermostatically controlled air temperatures between 40° and 120°C permit heat-sensitive materials to be dried. For small batches a hot air oven is, therefore, often the plant of choice. However, the following inherent limitations have led to the development of other small dryers:

a. A large floor space is required for the oven and tray loading facilities.
b. Labor costs for loading and unloading the oven are high.
c. Long drying times, usually about 24 hr, are necessary.
d. Solvents can be recovered from the air only with difficulty.
e. Unless carefully designed, nonuniform distribution of air over the trays gives variation in temperature and drying times within the oven. Variations of ±7°C in temperature have been found from location to location during the drying of tablet granules. Poor air circulation may permit local saturation and the cessation of drying.

If the material is of suitable granular form, drying times may be reduced to an hour or less by passing the air downward through the material laid on mesh trays. The oven in this form is called a batch-through-circulation dryer.

## 6.10.2 Vacuum Tray Dryers

Vacuum tray dryers [Figure 6.8(a)], differing only in size from the familiar laboratory vacuum oven, offer an alternative method for drying small quantities of material. When scaled up, construction becomes massive to withstand the applied vacuum and cost is further increased by the associated vacuum equipment. Vacuum tray dryers are, therefore, only used when a definite advantage over the hot air oven is secured, such as low-temperature drying of thermolabile materials or the recovery of solvents from the bed. The exclusion of oxygen may also be advantageous or necessary in some operations.

Heat is usually supplied by passing steam or hot water through hollow shelves. Drying temperatures can be carefully controlled and, for the major part of the drying cycle, the material remains at the boiling point of the wetting

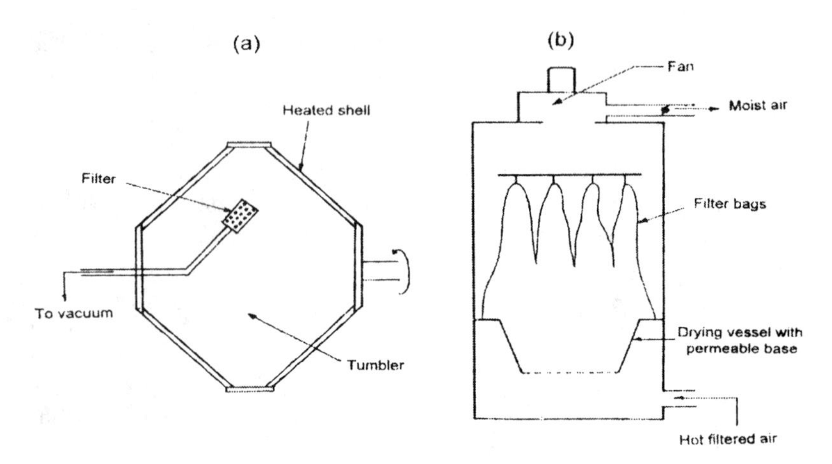


**FIGURE 6.8** (a) Rotary vacuum dryer and (b) fluidized bed dryer.

liquid under the operating vacuum. Radiation from the shelf above may cause a significant increase in temperature at the surface of the material if high drying temperatures are used. Drying times are long, usually about 12 to 48 hr.

### 6.10.3 Tumbling Dryers

The limitations of ovens, particularly with respect to the long drying times, has, where possible, promoted the design and application of other batch dryers. The simplest of these is the tumble dryer, for which the most common shape is the double cone in Figure 6.8(a). Operating under vacuum, this dryer provides controlled low-temperature drying, the possibility of solvent recovery, and increased rates of drying. Heat is supplied to the tumbling charge by contact with the heated shell and by heat transfer through the vapor. Optimum conditions are established experimentally by varying the vacuum, temperature, and, if the material passes through a sticky stage, rotation speed. With correct operation a uniform powder should be obtained, as distinct from the cakes produced when static beds are dried. Some materials, such as waxy solids, cannot be dried by this method because the tumbling action causes the material to aggregate into balls.

A normal charge would be about 60% of the total volume, and, for dryers 0.7 to 2 m in diameter, drying times of 2 to 12 hr may be expected. When applied to drying tablet granules, periods of 2 to 4 hr replace the 18 to 24 hr obtained with hot air ovens. The mixing and granulating capacity of the tumbling action has suggested that these operations could precede drying in the same apparatus.

## 6.10.4 Fluidized Bed Dryers

The term *fluidization* is applied to processes in which a loose, porous bed of solids is converted to a fluid system, having the properties of surface leveling, flow and pressure-depth relationships, by passing the fluid up through the bed.

Fluidized bed techniques, employing air as the fluidizing medium, have been successfully applied to drying when the solid is of suitable physical form. The high interfacial contact between drying air and solids gives drying rates 10 to 20 times greater than are obtained during tray drying. A drying curve for this method is shown in Figure 6.9.

The dryer, illustrated in Figure 6.8(b), consists of a basket of plastic or stainless steel with a perforated bottom mounted in the body of the drier and into which the material to be dried is placed. Heated air may be blown or sucked through the bed. The air leaving the basket passes through an air filter and may be recirculated. Particle properties, such as shape and size distribution, affect fluidization, and a unit must have a variable airflow, adjusted so that the material is fluidized but is not carried into the filters. For this reason, the material must have a fairly close size range or elutriation of fine particles into the filters will take place.

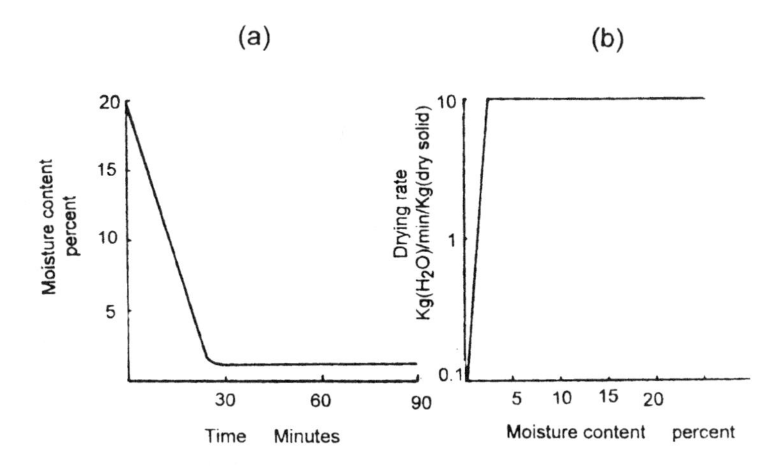


**FIGURE 6.9** Drying curves.

Fluidized bed dryers are particularly suitable for granulated materials and are increasingly being used for tablet granulations when product change-over is not too frequent. It may be advantageous to preform other materials, such as a dewatered filter cake, into granules solely in order to employ fluidized bed drying. If fluidizing conditions are ideal, the granulation will not require further grinding. Tray dryers, on the other hand, produce a caked product that may require mild comminution. Variation in temperature, which may be quite marked in tray dryers, is virtually eliminated in fluidized bed dryers by the intense mixing action. The floor space for a given capacity is small compared with a tray dryer. Machines vary in size, handling up to 250 kg. Drying times, maximum, minimum, and optimum air velocities, air temperature, and the tendency to cake and channel are established experimentally since they cannot be predicted accurately at present.

Considerable erosion and the production of large amounts of fines might be expected from the intense turbulent movement. Experience shows that the opposite is true. The particles are to some extent "padded" by the surrounding fluid so that either the amount of contact between particles is low or the impact energy is small.

### 6.10.5 Agitated Batch Dryers

Agitated batch dryers consist of a jacketed cylindrical vessel with agitator blades designed to scrape the bottom and the walls. The body may be run at atmospheric pressure or under vacuum. Pasty materials, which could not be handled in tumbling or fluidized bed dryers, may be successfully dried at rates higher than can be achieved in an oven.

### 6.10.6 Freeze-Drying

Freeze-drying is an extreme form of vacuum drying in which the solid is frozen and drying takes place by subliming the solid phase (Pikal et al., 1984; Nail, 1980; Jennings, 1988; Dushman and Lafferty, 1962). Low temperatures and pressures are used. Establishing and maintaining these conditions, together with the low drying rates obtained, create a most expensive method of drying which is only used on a large scale when other methods are inadequate.

Freeze-drying is extensively used in two principal fields: (1) when high rates of decomposition occur during normal drying; (2) with substances that can be dried at higher temperatures but are thereby changed in some way. Fruit juices, for example, are reputed to lose subtle elements of flavor and odor, and proteinaceous materials are partly denatured by the concentration and higher temperatures associated with conventional drying. Drying blood plasma and some antibiotics are important large-scale applications of freeze-drying. On a smaller scale, it is extensively used for the dehydration of bacteria, vaccines, blood fractions, and tissues.

Freeze-drying is theoretically a simple technique. Pure ice exhibits an equilibrium vapor pressure of 4.6 mmHg at 0°C and 0.1 mmHg at −40°C. The vapor pressure of ice containing dissolved substances will, of course, be lower. If, however, the pressure above the frozen solution is less than its equilibrium vapor pressure, the ice will sublime, eventually leaving the solute as a sponge-like residue equal in apparent volume to the original solid and, therefore, of low bulk density. The latter is readily dissolved when water is added, and freeze-drying has been called *lyophilic drying* or *lyophilization* for this reason. No concentration, in the normal sense of the word, occurs, and structural changes in, for example, protein solutions are minimized.

In practice, many difficulties are encountered. Under conditions of high vacuum, water vapor must be trapped or eliminated. To maintain drying, heat must be supplied to the frozen solid to balance the latent heat of sublimation without melting the solid. Difficulties become acute if, like blood plasma, the product is dried in the final container under aseptic conditions.

In the first stage of the process, the material is cooled and frozen. If the temperature of a dilute solution of a salt is slowly reduced, leveling occurs in the time-temperature curve just below 0°C, due to the liberation of the latent heat of fusion of ice, and pure ice separates. With further cooling, the solution becomes concentrated until the eutectic mixture is formed. This freezes to give a plateau in the cooling curve. It is a clear indication of complete freezing. If the concentration of the liquid eutectic mixture is small, the material may appear to be completely frozen at higher temperatures. Under these conditions, some drying from a liquid phase will occur, possibly with damaging results. This can be detected by measuring the electrical resistance of the ice, which becomes infinitely great when the eutectic mixture freezes. Conversely, thawing gives a marked decrease in resistance, an effect that can be used to automatically control the state of the drying solid. Protein solutions do not give clearly defined eutectic points and are usually frozen to below −25°C before drying. Freezing is carried out quickly to prevent concentration of the solution and to produce fine ice crystals. Some degree of supercooling may be induced followed by a very quick freeze. Freezing may or may not be carried out in the drying chamber. If drying in final containers is necessary, small-scale operations may employ immersion in a coolant such as liquid air or isopentane. Larger-scale installations may cool with a blast of very cold air. Alternatively, evaporative freezing, in which the liquid is cooled to near its freezing point and the system rapidly evacuated, is employed. The evaporating liquid cools and freezes rapidly. Frothing caused by the evolution of dissolved gases may complicate this technique. For bulk drying the liquid is placed in shallow trays on refrigerated shelves in the drying cabinet.

A suitable ratio of surface area to depth of solid must be provided to facilitate drying. Thin layers of frozen liquid are used in bulk drying. The surface area of bottle-dried plasma may be increased by spinning in a vertical axis during freezing to give a frozen shell about 2 cm thick around the inside periphery of the bottle. Spinning also prevents frothing during evaporative freezing by inhibiting the formation of bubbles.

In plasma processing, freezing, and drying, handling must be carried out aseptically. This is maintained by a filter at the neck of the bottle that allows the passage of water vapor but prevents the ingress of bacteria. Similar precautions are taken during the drying of antibiotics.

Effective drying vacuum of from 0.05 to 0.2 mmHg may be provided by directly pumping water vapor and permanent gases, originally present or derived from the drying material and from leaks, out of the system. Normal practice, however, favors interposing a refrigerated condenser between the drying surface and the pump. This arrangement allows a smaller pump, handling mainly permanent gases, to be used but demands a low condenser temperature, such as −50°C, to remove water vapor at the low operating pressure. A system for bulk drying in trays is represented in Figure 6.10(a).

During drying, heat must be supplied to the drying surface. When drying a material, such as plasma, in a final container, a temperature gradient is established across the container wall and through the ice to the drying surface by

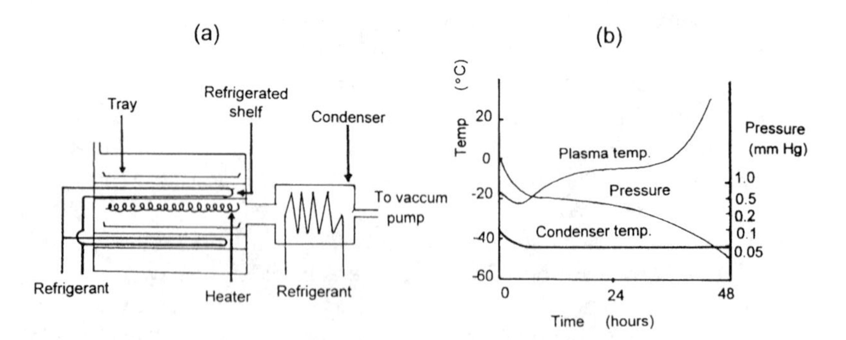


**FIGURE 6.10** (a) Equipment for freeze-drying bulk liquids in trays and (b) variations in temperature and pressure during the freeze-drying cycle for blood plasma.

means of a heater suitably mounted in relation to the container. The power dissipated by the heater must be carefully controlled so that melting does not occur at the ice-container junction, the point nearest the heat source and at highest temperature. At any time, the prevailing conditions are such that the evaporation rate is approximately constant and temperatures and pressure adjust so that there are temperature and pressure gradients from the drying surface to the condenser. As evaporation proceeds, a drying line recedes into the solid. With the thinning of the ice layer, the temperature gradient through the ice will be modified by the decreasing resistance to heat flow. An increase in the rate of drying due to increase in temperature and vapor pressure of the drying surface might, therefore, be expected. In practice, this increase is modified by the layer of dried plasma, which offers considerable resistance to the flow of vapor. The bacterial filter also causes a large, constant pressure drop. Evaporation of pure ice without the filter and plasma layer would be 300 times faster. When the plasma is nearly dry, its temperature is allowed to rise to about 30°C to facilitate final drying. The total drying time is about 48 hr. The temperatures and pressure in the system during this period are shown, as a function of time, in Figure 6.10(b).

If the product is not being dried in its final container, radiant heat may be used to provide the latent heat of sublimation. If the dried solid could be removed continuously, high drying rates are possible. Not only is heat provided directly to the drying surface but also there is little danger of melting the ice at the container wall.

## 6.11 CONTINUOUS DRYERS

Although many types of continuous dryers are available, the scale of the operation for which they are designed is rarely appropriate to pharmaceutical manufacture. As with most continuous plant items, the cost is disproportionately high for small units. Spray and drum dryers provide an exception to this comment because residence times in the dryers are short and thermal degradation is minimized. Under some conditions, freeze-drying may be the only practical alternative.

### 6.11.1 Spray Dryers

As the name implies, the solution or suspension to be dried is sprayed into a hot airstream and circulated through a chamber. The dried product may be

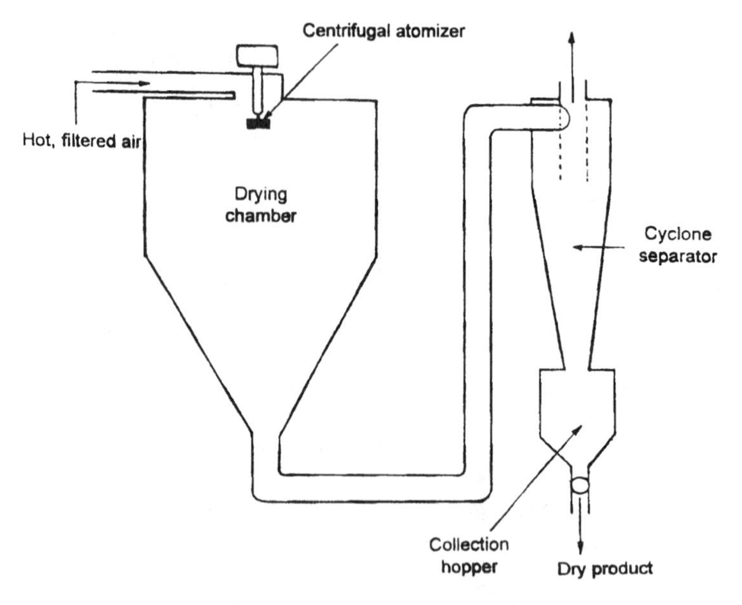


**FIGURE 6.11** Spray dryer.

carried out to a cyclone or bag separator or may fall to the bottom of the drying chamber and be expelled through a valve. The chambers are normally cylindrical with a conical bottom, although proportions vary widely. A typical spray dryer is illustrated in Figure 6.11.

The process can be divided into four sections: fluid atomization, mixing the droplets, drying, and removing and collecting the dry particles. Atomization may be achieved by means of single fluid or two fluid nozzles or by spinning disk atomizers. The single fluid nozzle [Figure 6.12(a)] operates by forcing the solution under pressure through a fine hole into the airstream. An intense swirl is conferred on the liquid before it emerges from the orifice. This causes the jet to break up. In the two fluid nozzles [Figure 6.12(b)] a jet of air simultaneously emerges from an annular aperture concentric with the liquid orifice. Both types are subject to clogging and severe erosion, so neither is well suited to spraying suspensions. The spinning disks [Figure 6.12(c)] are most versatile and consist, in their simplest form, of a mushroom-shaped disk spinning at 5000 to 30,000 rpm. Other designs include the slotted disk [Figure 6.12(d)] which will spray thick suspensions and, if special feeding arrangements are used, pastes. The main factors that determine droplets size are the liquid's viscosity and surface tension, the fluid pressure in the nozzles, or, for

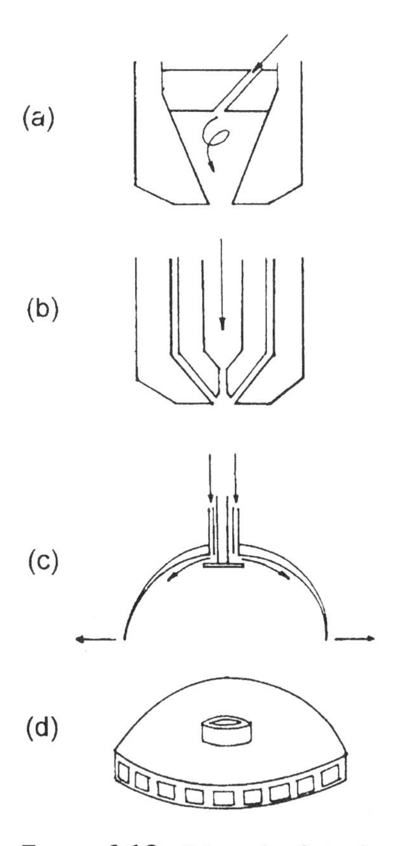


**FIGURE 6.12** Schematic of atomizers for spray drying.

spinning disks, their size and speed of rotation. A reasonably uniform and controllable size within the range 10–500 μm is desirable.

In vertical spray dryers, the flow of the drying gas may be concurrent or countercurrent with respect to the movement of droplets. The movement of the gas is, however, complex and highly turbulent. Good mixing of droplets and gas occurs, and the heat and mass transfer rates are high. In conjunction with the large interfacial area conferred by atomization, these factors give very high evaporation rates. The residence time of a droplet in the dryer is only a few seconds (5–30 s). Since the material is at wet bulb temperature for much of this time, high gas temperatures of 150–200°C may be used even with thermolabile materials. Although the temperature of the material rises above the wet bulb temperature at the end of the process, the drying gases will be cooler and the material will be almost dry, a condition in which many materials are thermally less sensitive. For these reasons it is possible to dry complex vegetable extracts, such as coffee or digitalis, milk products, spore suspensions, and other labile materials without significant loss of potency or flavor.

Drying is considered to take place by simple evaporation rather than by boiling, and it has been observed that a droplet reaches a terminal velocity within about 30 cm of the atomizer. Beyond this, there is no relative velocity between the droplet and the drying gas unless the former is very large. The droplets may dry to form a solid, spherical particle. If, however, the emerging solids form a skin, internal pressure may inflate the particle and the final dry form will be hollow spheres that may or may not have a blowhole. These xenospheres may also fragment, so the final product occurs as agglomerates of finely divided solids. It has been found experimentally that the product's bulk density, which is lowest for xenospheres and highest for fragmented solids, increases as the inlet air temperature is lowered and as the droplet size increases. A higher feed concentration also increases the bulk density because drops of the same size give spheres with thicker walls.

These attractive physical characteristics lend further advantage to spray-drying. The product often has excellent flow and packing properties that greatly facilitate handling and transport. As an example, spray-dried lactose is a widely used tablet excipient which will flow, pack, and compact without prior granulation. Similarly, a slurry of fillers and other excipients could be granulated by spraying and drying. After adding an active principle, the mix could be compressed without further processing.

The capital and running costs of spray dryers are high, but if the scale is sufficiently large it may provide the cheapest method. When thermolabile materials are dried on a small scale, costs will be 10 to 20 times greater than for oven drying. Air used to dry fine chemicals or food products is heated indirectly, thus reducing thermal efficiency and increasing costs. In some other installations, hot gases from combustion may be used directly.

### 6.11.2 Drum Dryers

The drum dryer consists of one or two slowly rotating, steam-heated cylinders. These are coated with solution or slurry by means of a dip feed, illustrated in Figure 6.13. The lower portion of the drum is immersed in an agitated trough of feed material or, in the case of some double-drum dryers, by feeding

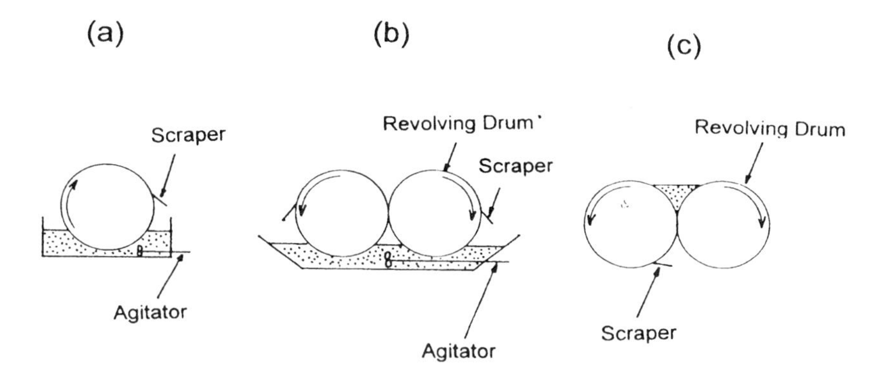


**FIGURE 6.13** Drum dryers.

the liquor into the gap between the cylinders as shown in Figure 6.13. Spray and splash feeds are also used. When dip feeding is employed, the hot drum must not boil the liquid in the trough. Drying takes place by simple evaporation rather than by boiling. The dried material is scraped from the drum at a suitable point by a knife.

Drying capacity is influenced by drum speed and feed temperature. The latter may be preheated. With the double-drum dryer, the gap between the cylinders determines the film thickness.

Drum dryers, like spray dryers, are relatively expensive in small sizes and their use in the pharmaceutical industry is largely confined to drying thermolabile materials where the short contact time is advantageous. Drums are normally fabricated from stainless or chrome-plated steel to reduce contamination. The heat treatment to which the solid is subjected is greater than in spray-drying and the physical form of the product is often less attractive. During drying, the liquid approaches its boiling point and the dry solids approach the temperature of the drum surface.

# 7

# Solid-Liquid Extraction

Leaching or solid-liquid extraction are terms used to describe the extraction of soluble constituents from a solid or semisolid by means of suitable solvents. The process, which is used domestically whenever tea or coffee is made, is an important stage in the production of many fine chemicals found naturally in animal and vegetable tissue. Examples are found in the extraction of fixed oils from seeds, this method offering an alternative to mechanical expression, in the preparation of alkaloids, such as strychnine from *Nux vomica* beans or quinine from *Cinchona* bark, and in the isolation of enzymes, such as renin, and hormones, such as insulin, from animal sources. In the past, a wider importance attended the process because the products of simple extraction procedures, known as Galenicals, formed the major part of the ingredients used to fulfill a doctor's prescription.

## 7.1 METHODS OF LEACHING

Leaching in the pharmaceutical and allied industries is operated as a batch process. This is because high-cost materials are processed in relatively small quantities. Frequent changes of material may be made, creating problems of cleaning and contamination. For these reasons, continuous extraction, which is characterized by a large throughput and the mechanical movement of the solid counter to the flow of solvent, is not applicable to pharmaceutical extraction and is not described in this text.

Whatever the scale of the extraction, however, leaching is performed in one of two ways. In the first, the raw material is placed in a vessel, forming a permeable bed through which the solvent or menstruum percolates. Dissolution of the wanted constituents occurs and the solution issues from the bottom of the bed. This liquid is sometimes called the *miscella*, and the exhausted solids are called the *marc*. This process will be called *leaching by percolation*. The alternative process is *leaching by immersion* and consists of immersing the solid in the solvent and stirring. After a suitable period of time, solid and liquid are separated.

## 7.2 LEACHING BY PERCOLATION

Coarse ground material is placed in the body of the extractor. This may be jacketed to give control of the extraction temperature. The packing must be even or the solvent will preferentially flow through a limited volume of the bed and leaching will be inefficient. In large extractors, channeling is prevented or reduced by horizontal, perforated plates placed at intervals in the bed. These redistribute the percolating liquid.

Solvent inhibition will swell dried materials and the permeability of the bed will be reduced. This is most marked with aqueous solvents. If swelling occurs, it is necessary to moisten the material with water or with the solvent before it is packed into the extractor.

Once the extractor is packed, leaching may be conducted in a number of ways. The body of the extractor may be completely filled with the solvent. Liquid is then withdrawn from the body through the false bottom and more solvent is added. This is continued until the marc is exhausted. Alternatively, the solution issuing from the bottom may be returned to the top. After a period of recirculation, the liquid is completely withdrawn and fresh solvent admitted. In both processes, a period of steeping or soaking may precede the movement of liquid.

In beds of high permeability, adequate liquid movement is obtained by simple gravity operation in an open vessel. If the material forms a dense bed, however, the liquid must be pumped through if suitable flow rates are to be secured. A closed extraction vessel must then be used. Closed extraction vessels are also necessary for high-temperature extraction and extraction with volatile solvents. In alternative methods the liquid is forced upward through the bed. Possible migration of fine material downward and the formation of a region of low permeability at the bottom of the bed are prevented in this way. In other processes, the bed may not be immersed in the menstruum. This is simply sprinkled onto the upper surface and allowed to trickle through the bed, the voids of which are mainly filled with air.

Simple extractions of this type, if carried to completion, require large amounts of solvent and yield dilute extracts. These disadvantages can be overcome if extraction is followed by evaporation. These operations are often integrated in extraction plant. The leach liquids leaving the extractor enter an evaporator heated, for example, by a calandria. Since most materials encountered are heat sensitive, the evaporator is operated at reduced pressure. The vapor leaving the evaporator is condensed and returned to the extractor. When extraction is carried out with water-immiscible solvents, any water derived from the feed material and present in the condensate is separated and rejected. The extraction is stopped when the leach liquid is free from wanted constituents. A concentrated extract remains in the evaporator.

Leaching by percolation provides a simple method of separating leach liquid and solid during the extraction. When this is complete, the permeable bed largely drains, permitting extensive solvent recovery. Further recovery can be gained by mechanical expression.

## 7.3 LEACHING BY IMMERSION

In pharmaceutical processes, leaching by immersion is carried out in simple tanks which may be agitated by a turbine or paddle. If the solids are adequately suspended, intimate contact between the phases promotes efficient extraction. Incomplete extraction due to channeling is avoided and difficulties due to swelling do not arise. Problems arise, however, in the subsequent separation of the phases. The materials to which leaching by immersion is applied are normally finely divided or coarse and compressible. When agitation ceases, the solids settle and the leach liquid can be siphoned or pumped off by lines suitably placed in the tank. The sediment, however, contains a large volume of the leach liquid which must be recovered by resuspending the solids in fresh solvent, allowing the solids to sediment, and decanting the supernatant liquid. Cake filtration provides an alternative method of separation. The leach liquid remaining in the cake is displaced by passing a wash liquid. In some cases, a filter press may be used for extraction and separation.

## 7.4 THE CHOICE OF EXTRACTION METHOD

The choice of extraction method depends primarily on the physical properties of the basic material and its particle size. If this material is a coarse, rigid powder, beds of high permeability will form and percolation can be adopted. The expense of finer grinding is avoided, and the subsequent separation of solids and liquid is facilitated. The process can be conducted in such a way that a concentrated product is obtained. Other materials, such as fine powders or compressible animal tissues, will not form permeable beds, and the alternative method must be adopted. Some compensation for the difficulties of separation and the dilution of the extract during washing may be found in a more rapid and more complete extraction, due to the use of finer powders, the intimate contact between solids and liquid, and the absence of channeling.

The use of pressure extends the application of percolation to materials which form beds of low permeability. Alternatively, permeability may be increased by grinding the solids with a supporting material such as glass wool.

## 7.5 THE CHOICE OF SOLVENT

The ideal solvent is cheap, nontoxic, and noninflammable. It is highly selective, dissolving only the wanted constituents of the solid. It should have a low viscosity, allowing easy movement through a bed of solids, and, if the resulting solution is to be concentrated by evaporation, a high vapor pressure. These factors greatly limit the number of solvents of commercial value. Water and alcohol, and mixtures of the two, are widely used. Both, however, are nonselective, leaching varying proportions of gums, mucilages, and other unwanted components. Most of the tinctures and liquid extracts used in pharmacy are simple, impure extracts made with water or mixtures of water and alcohol. Acidified or alkaline mixtures of water and alcohol are used to extract insulin from minced pancreas. A more selective extraction is given by petroleum solvents and benzene and related solvents. In the preparation of many pure alkaloids, the powdered material is moistened with an alkaline solution, packed into a bed, and leached with petroleum. Subsequent purification by fractional crystallization is facilitated by the absence of gums. Acetone and chlorinated hydrocarbons also find applications in leaching. In some cases, specific properties of the wanted constituents may suggest a particular solvent. Eugenol, for example, can be readily extracted from cloves with a solution of potassium hydroxide. Care must be given to the selection of solvents, because they may be subject to regulatory control due to their toxicity or impact on the environment.

## 7.6 FACTORS AFFECTING THE RATE OF LEACHING

Whatever method is adopted, leaching consists of a number of consecutive diffusional or mass transfer processes. The solvent first penetrates the raw material, and the soluble elements dissolve. These diffuse in the opposite direction to the surface of the solid matrix and then through the liquid layers at its surface to reach the bulk solution. These processes proceed under the influence of an overall concentration gradient, the concentration being least in the bulk solution. Any of these processes may be responsible for limiting the rate at which leaching proceeds. In pharmaceutical leaching, however, the solid matrix is usually cellular, which normally offers the highest diffusional resistance. The complexity of such structures does not permit a strict analysis of the mass transfer processes. Nevertheless, the simple diffusional concepts expressed in Fick's law suggest that the following factors influence the rate of leaching: the size distribution of the leached particles, the temperature of leaching, the physical properties of solvent, and the relative movement imposed upon the solids and the liquid.

## 7.7 SIZE AND SIZE DISTRIBUTION OF THE SOLID PARTICLES

The particle size of the solids determines the distance which solvent and solute must diffuse within the solid matrix. Since this offers the major diffusional resistance, reduction of the distance by comminution greatly increases the leaching rate, the concentration gradient being effectively increased. In addition, the inverse relationship between particle size and surface area prescribes an increase in the area of contact between the matrix and the surrounding liquid. Solute transfer at this boundary is therefore facilitated. In leaching by immersion, a further advantage conferred by size reduction is the ease with which finer particles are suspended. Finally, extensive cell rupture occurs during grinding, allowing more direct contact between solvent and solute and more rapid dissolution and diffusion.

Other factors, however, operate against size reduction. Leaching by percolation demands formation of a permeable bed. Low permeability gives low flow rates and low rates of extraction. Permeability is a complex function of particle size and porosity, the former determining how a given void space is to be disposed within the bed. The disposition of the void space consists of a few channels of relatively large diameter, i.e., a bed of high permeability, if the particle size is large. In leaching by immersion, the difficulties of separating solid and liquid increase as the particle size decreases.

The opposition of the factors suggests an optimum particle size for any extraction. This is determined to some extent by the physical nature of the solids. A dense, woody structure would be extracted as a fine powder. An example is given by the root of *Ipecacuanha*. A leafy structure, on the other hand, would be more satisfactorily leached as a coarse powder.

Porosity and permeability are influenced by the particle size distribution. A high porosity is secured if the distribution is narrow. Small particles may otherwise fill the interstices created by the contact of larger particles. After grinding, therefore, it is often necessary to classify the product and remove undersize material, which is then bulked with the fines from other batches and separately extracted. A further advantage arising from a narrow size distribution is even packing and the creation of a regular system of pores and waists. This promotes even movement of solvent and solution through the bed.

In some cases, size reduction may take a particular form. Seeds and beans are often rolled or flaked to produce extensive cell rupture. In other processes, the cell wall, although depressing the rate of extraction, may make the extraction more selective by preventing the movement of unwanted materials of high molecular weight. Here, the size reduction must leave most cells intact.

## 7.8 TEMPERATURE

Within the limits imposed by the thermal stability of the wanted constituents, a high extraction temperature appears desirable. The solubility of most materials increases as the temperature increases, so higher solute concentrations and higher concentration gradients are possible. The increased solubility and increased diffusivity give higher extraction rates. In very many cases, however, materials are susceptible to heat degradation, and cold extraction must be used.

In addition, the selectivity of a solvent may be impaired at high temperatures. An example of the use of moderately high temperatures is the extraction of *Rauwolfia* alkaloids with boiling methanol.

## 7.9 PHYSICAL PROPERTIES OF THE SOLVENT

The relevant properties of the solvent are low viscosity and free solution of wanted constituents. These properties, along with other aspects of the solvent, have already been discussed.

## 7.10 RELATIVE MOVEMENT IMPOSED ON THE SOLIDS AND THE LIQUID

The major and controlling resistance to solute diffusion to the bulk solution is normally found in the cell matrix. Increased rate of movement of the solution past the surface will not, therefore, greatly affect the extraction rate, in marked contrast to the processes of dissolution and crystallization. Nevertheless, movement is imposed on the menstruum in both general methods described.

In the percolation of a liquid through a bed of solids, mass transfer of the solute from the surfaces of the solid to the liquid in the interstices of the bed takes place by molecular diffusion and by natural convection arising from the density changes created by dissolution. Although these processes are slow, they are much quicker than mass transfer in the matrix under the same differences in concentration. Concentration gradients in the liquid outside the particles are, therefore, very low. At any point in the bed, the introduction of dilute solution from above and the loss of concentrated solution to below decreases the interstitial concentration by dilution or displacement. This effect can be considered simply to decrease the solute concentration at the junction of solid and solution, thus imposing a favorable concentration gradient within the matrix.

Similarly, the agitation of the slurry in leaching by immersion is not primarily to decrease the boundary layer thickness at the surface and its diffusional resistance. Rather, agitation serves only to keep the particles in suspension and to equalize the solute concentration throughout the liquid. If the particles settle, the solute must diffuse through the stagnant fluid filling the interstices of the bed. High diffusional resistance is created and the rate of extraction is depressed.

# 8

# Crystallization

As a unit operation, the term *crystallization* describes the production of a solid, single-component, crystalline phase from a multicomponent fluid phase. It may be applied to the production of crystalline solids from vapors, melts, or solutions. Crystallization from solution is most important. To complete the preparation of a pure dry solid, it is also necessary to separate the solid from the fluid phase. This is usually carried out by centrifugation or filtration and by drying. The importance of crystallization lies primarily in the purification achieved during the process and in the physical properties of the product. A crystalline powder is easily handled, is stable, and often possesses good flow properties and an attractive appearance.

Crystallization from a vapor, which occurs naturally, for example, in the formation of hoarfrost, is employed in sublimation processes and for the condensation of water vapor during freeze-drying. Equipment may be regarded as specialized condensers in which the principal problems are removal of the latent heat of crystallization and discharge of the solid condensate. Condensers are commonly mounted in parallel so that one can be shut down and emptied manually, by conveyor or by melting and draining, without interrupting sublimation. This process is not further considered.

In the pharmaceutical industry, crystallization is usually performed on a small scale from solutions, often in jacketed or agitated vessels. The conditions of crystallization, necessary for suitable purity, yield, and crystal form, are usually established by experiment. Nevertheless a study of the principal factors which control crystallization is important. In this study, much information is derived from the behavior of carefully prepared melts. These reveal more clearly than solutions the two stages of crystallization: nucleation and crystal growth. Nucleation describes the formation of small nuclei around which crystals grow. Without the formation of nuclei, crystal growth cannot occur.

## 8.1 CRYSTALLIZATION IN MELTS

A melt may be defined as the liquid form of a single material or the homogeneous liquid form of two or more materials which solidifies on cooling. Crystallization in such a system is described by the following sequence: imposition of supercooling, formation of nuclei, and crystal growth.

If a single-component liquid is cooled, some degree, often large, of supercooling must be established before crystal nuclei are formed and growth begins. A metastable liquid region exists below the melting point, which can only be entered by cooling. In this metastable, supercooled region, the absence of nucleation precludes the formation and growth of crystals. If, however, a crystal seed is added, growth occurs. The deliberate seeding of a metastable system is commonly employed in industrial crystallization. With further cooling, spontaneous nucleation usually takes place and the released heat of crystallization raises the temperature of the melt to its true melting point. With some materials, lower temperatures increase the viscosity and prevent nucleation. The liquid then solidifies into a mass without crystallizing, a process known as *vitrification*, the products of which are called *glasses*. Many organic materials can be obtained in this form, and, as with glass itself, devitrification may suddenly occur, particularly after heating.

## 8.2 NUCLEATION

In certain single-component systems, such as piperidine, nucleation and crystal growth are independent and can be separately studied. The rate of nucleation as a function of supercooling is studied by maintaining the melt, for a certain time, at the given temperature and then quickly raising the temperature to the

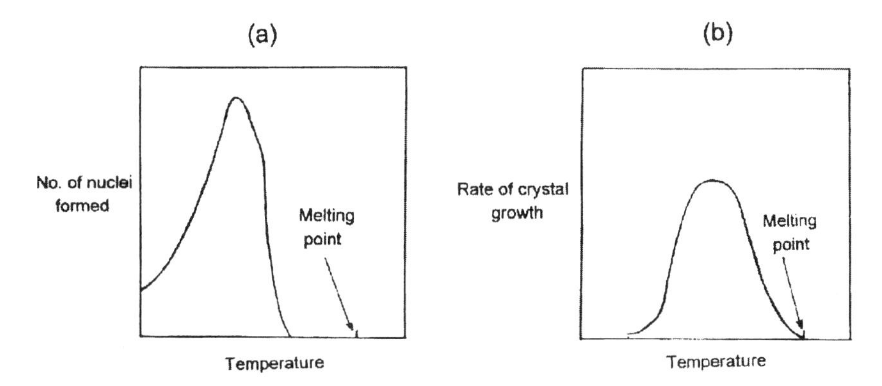


**FIGURE 8.1** (a) Change in nucleation with degree of supercooling; (b) change in rate of crystal growth with degree of supercooling.

metastable region where further nucleation is negligible but the already formed nuclei can grow. Figure 8.1(a) describes the results of such an experiment. At low degrees of supercooling little or no nucleation takes place. With further cooling, the rate of nucleation rises to a maximum and then falls. The relation therefore indicates that excessive cooling may depress the rate of crystallization by limiting the number of nuclei formed.

Spontaneous nucleation is considered to occur when sufficient molecules of low kinetic energy come together in such a way that the attraction between them is sufficient to overcome their momentum. The growth of a nucleus probably takes place over a very short time in a region of high local concentration. Once a certain size is reached, the nucleus stabilizes in the prevailing conditions. As the temperature falls, more low-energy molecules are present and the nucleation rate rises. The decrease in nucleation rate at lower temperature is due to increased melt viscosity.

## 8.3 CRYSTAL GROWTH

If nucleation and crystal growth are independent, the latter can be studied by seeding a melt with small crystals in conditions of little or no natural nucleation. The growth rate can then be measured. The relation between growth rate and temperature [Figure 8.1(b)] also exhibits an optimal degree of supercooling, although the maximum growth temperature is normally higher than the temperature of maximum nucleation. The form of the crystal growth curve is again explained by the molecular kinetics. At temperatures just below the melting point, molecules have too much energy to remain in the crystal lattice. As the temperature falls, more molecules are retained and the growth rate increases. Ultimately, however, diffusion to and orientation at the crystal surface are depressed.

For crystal growth in a single-component melt, the molecules at the crystal surface must reach the correct position at the lattice and become suitably orientated, thereby losing kinetic energy. These energy changes appear as heat of crystallization, and this heat must be transferred from the surface to the bulk of the melt. The crystal growth rate is influenced by the heat transfer rate and the changes taking place at the surface. Agitation of the system increases heat transfer by reducing the thermal resistance of the liquid layers adjacent to the crystal until the changes at the crystal face become the controlling effect.

In multicomponent melts and solutions, material deposition at the crystal face depletes the adjacent liquid layers and a concentration gradient is set up with saturation at the face and supersaturation in the liquid. Diffusion of molecules to the crystal face is discussed in the next section.

The foregoing account describes the behavior of certain carefully prepared melts from which all extraneous matter is rigidly excluded. Dust and other insoluble matter may increase the nucleation rate by acting as centers of crystallization. Soluble impurities may increase or decrease the rates of nucleation and crystal growth. The latter is probably due to adsorption of the impurity on the crystal face. Impurities may also affect the form in which the material crystallizes.

## 8.4 CRYSTALLIZATION FROM SOLUTIONS

When a material crystallizes from a solution, nucleation and crystal growth occur simultaneously over a wide intermediate temperature range, so a study of these processes is more difficult. In general, however, they are thought to be similar to nucleation and crystal growth in melts. The three basic steps—induction of supersaturation, formation of nuclei, and crystals growth—are explained with reference to the solubility curve in Figure 8.2.

A solution with temperature and concentration indicated by point A may be saturated by cooling to point B or by removing solvent (point C). With further cooling or concentration, the supersaturated metastable region is entered. If the degree of supersaturation is small, then spontaneous formation of crystal nuclei is highly improbable. Crystal growth, however, can occur if

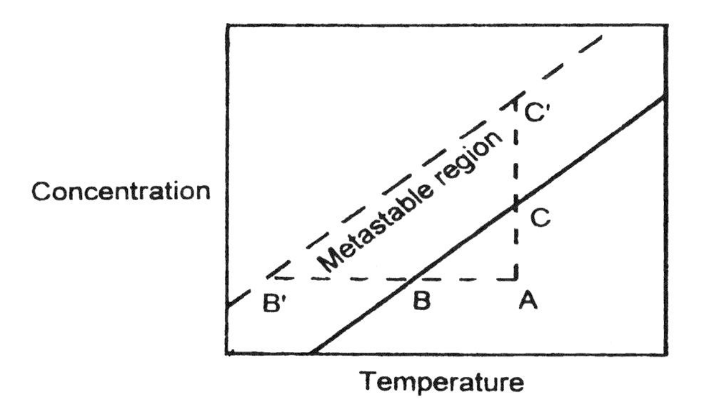


**FIGURE 8.2** Solubility-supersolubility diagram.

seeds are added. With greater supersaturation, spontaneous nucleation becomes more probable, and the metastable region is limited approximately by the line B′C′. If the solution is cooled to B′ or concentrated by solvent removal to C′, spontaneous nucleation is virtually certain. Crystal growth also occurs in these conditions. The growth rate, however, is depressed at low temperatures.

During crystal growth, deposition on the crystal faces causes depletion of molecules in the immediate vicinity. The driving force is provided by the concentration gradient set up from supersaturation in the solution to lower concentrations at the crystal face. A large degree of supersaturation therefore promotes a high growth rate. A reaction at the surface, in which solute molecules become correctly oriented in the crystal lattice, provides a second resistance to crystal growth. Simultaneously, the heat of crystallization must be conducted away.

Agitation modifies the rate of crystal growth for given conditions of temperature and saturation. Initially, agitation quickly increases the growth rate by decreasing the boundary layer thickness and the diffusional resistance. However, as agitation is intensified, a limiting value is reached which is determined by the kinetics of the surface reaction. In Figure 8.3, the effect of agitation on the crystal growth rate in solutions of sodium thiosulfate of differing degrees of supersaturation is described.

As with melts, soluble impurities may increase or retard the rate of nucleation. Insoluble materials may act as nuclei and promote crystallization. Impurities may also affect crystal form and, in some cases, are deliberately added to secure a product with good appearance, absence of caking, or suitable flow properties.

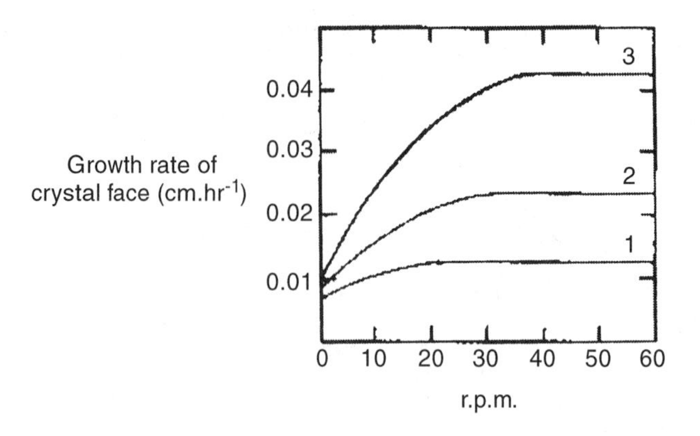


**FIGURE 8.3** Effect of agitation on growth rate of a sodium thiosulfate crystal.

The temperature at which crystallization is performed may be determined by the crystal form or degree of hydration required of the products. The solubility curves in Figure 8.4 show that crystallization at 50°C yields $FeSO_4{\cdot}7H_2O$; at 60°C, $FeSO_4{\cdot}4H_2O$; and at 70°C, $FeSO_4$. The majority of materials, however, have one or possibly two forms. The degree of supersaturation of solution 1 is 5 g/L, of solution 2 is 10 g/L, and of solution 3 is 15 g/L.

## 8.5 PRINCIPLES UNDERLYING THE DESIGN AND OPERATION OF CRYSTALLIZERS

The purpose of a crystallization plant is to produce, as far as possible, crystals of the required shape, size distribution, purity, and yield. This purpose is achieved by maintaining a degree of supersaturation at which nucleation and crystal growth proceed at appropriate rates. The number of nuclei formed controls the size of the crystals deposited from a given quantity of solution. Alternatively, crystal number and size can be controlled by adding the correct amount of artificial nuclei or seeds to a system in which little or no natural nucleation is taking place.

In most cases, the mode of operation is determined by the relation between the solubility of the solute and the temperature, examples of which are shown in Figure 8.4. This determines how supersaturation is to be achieved. Other factors of importance are the thermal stability of the solute, the impuri-

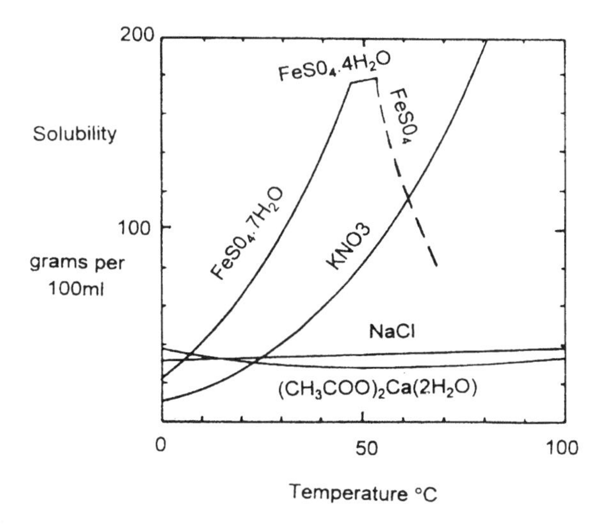


**FIGURE 8.4** Solubility curves.

ties which may be present, and the degree of hydration required. If the solubility of the solute increases greatly with temperature, supersaturation and the deposition of a large proportion of the solute is brought about by cooling a hot concentrated solution. Sodium nitrate provides an example. Sodium chloride and calcium acetate, on the other hand, exemplify materials with a small or negative temperature coefficient of solubility. Here, supersaturation can best be achieved by evaporating part of the solvent. In some cases, evaporation and cooling are employed. The mother liquors following evaporative crystallization can be cooled to yield a further crop of crystals, provided there is a suitable change in solubility and impurities present do not prohibit the process. In other crystallizers, flash cooling is used. A hot solution is passed into a vacuum chamber in which both evaporation and cooling take place.

Supersaturation can also be induced by the addition of a third substance which reduces the solubility of a solute in a solvent. These precipitation processes, which are important in the processing of thermolabile materials, are controlled by the mixing temperature, the agitation, and the rate at which the third substance is added. Water-insoluble materials dissolved in water-miscible organic solvents can be precipitated by adding water. Alternatively, the aqueous solubility of many materials can be reduced by the change of pH or by adding a common ion. Proteins can be salted out of solution by adding ammonium chloride and adjusting the pH. Finally, precipitation of a crystalline solid may be the result of a chemical reaction.

A crystallizer should produce crystals of uniform particle size, to facilitate removal of the mother liquor and washing. If large quantities of the liquor are occluded in the mass of crystals, drying yields an impure product. In addition, crystals of even size are less likely to cake on storage.

## 8.6 PRODUCTION OF VERY FINE CRYSTALS

Fine powders are important components in pharmaceutical operations. If a substance has a steep solubility curve, fine crystals are produced by quickly cooling the solution through the metastable region to conditions in which the nucleation rate is high and the crystal growth rate is low. This method is not always possible, and the precipitation methods described may be adopted.

## 8.7 PRODUCTION OF LARGE CRYSTALS

Batch production of large, uniform crystals may be carried out in agitated reaction vessels by slow controlled or natural cooling. Spontaneous nucleation is improbable until solution A is cooled to X. Crystallization then follows path XB. Better control is gained if the solution is artificially seeded. Seeding is shown at X′. Crystallization then follows the broken line X′B, the aim being to maintain the solution in the metastable region where growth rate is high and natural nucleation is low. The course of the crystallization is shown in Figure 8.5. Initially spontaneous nucleation may be allowed by cooling from

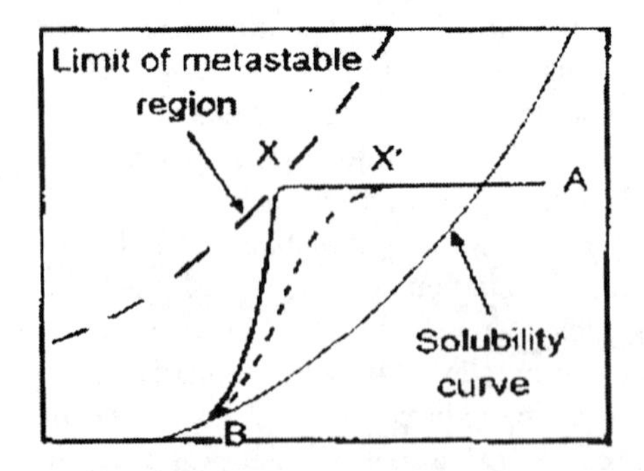


**FIGURE 8.5** Production of large crystals. The conditions of supersaturation.

A to X. As crystallization takes place, the degree of supersaturation and the concentration of the solute fall, ultimately reaching saturation at B when growth ceases. Closer control is secured by artificially seeding the supersaturated solution in conditions of no natural nucleation. Seeding is indicated by the point X′. The course of the crystallization is then indicated by the broken line X′B.

An important principle for the continuous production of large even crystals is used in Oslo or Krystal crystallizers. A metastable, supersaturated solution is released into the bottom of a mass of growing crystals on which the solute is deposited. The crystals are fluidized by the circulation of the solution, and classification in this zone allows the withdrawal of sufficiently large crystals from the bottom.

## 8.8 CRYSTALLIZERS

Although other methods may be adopted, crystallizers can be conveniently classified by the way in which a solution is supersaturated. This leads to the self-explanatory terms cooling crystallizer and evaporative crystallizer. In vacuum crystallizers, evaporation and cooling are used.

### 8.8.1 Cooling Crystallizers

Open or closed tanks, agitated by stirrers, are used for batch crystallization. The specific heat of the solution and the heat of crystallization are removed by means of jackets or coils through which cooling water can be circulated. Agitation destroys temperature gradients in the tanks, opposes sedimentation and irregular crystal growth at the bottom of the vessel, and, as described, facilitates growth. Similar equipment is used for crystallization or precipitation by adding a third substance.

Crystallizers for continuous processes often take the form of a trough cooled naturally or by a jacket. The solution enters at one end and crystals and liquid are discharged at the other. In one type of crystallizer, a slow-moving worm works in the solution and lifts crystals off the cooling surface to shower them through the solution and slowly convey them through the trough. The trough of another is agitated by rocking. Baffles are used to increase the residence time of the solution. Both crystallizers are characterized by low heat transfer coefficients, and an alternative arrangement consists essentially of a double-pipe heat exchanger. The crystallizing fluid is carried in

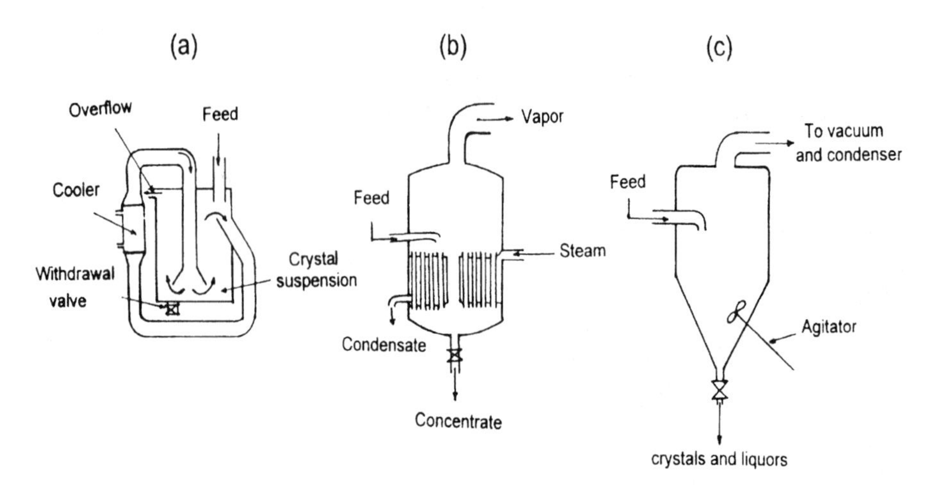


**FIGURE 8.6** (a) Cooling crystallizer; (b) evaporative crystallizer; (c) batch vacuum crystallizer.

the central pipe with countercurrent flow of the coolant in the annulus between the pipes. A shaft rotates in the central tube carrying blades which scrape the heat transfer surface. High heat transfer coefficients are obtained. An Oslo crystallizer, in which supersaturation is given by cooling, is described in Figure 8.6(a). The principles underlying this plant have already been described.

### 8.8.2 Evaporative Crystallizers

On a small scale, simple pans and stirred reaction vessels can be used for evaporative crystallization. Larger units may employ calandria heating, as shown in Figure 8.6(b). The downcomer, which must be large enough to accommodate the flow of the suspension, commonly houses an impeller, forced circulation increasing the heat transfer to the boiling liquid. These units may be adapted for batch or continuous processes in which crystal size is not of great importance. For continuous processes demanding close control of product size, an Oslo crystallizer which saturates the solution by evaporation may be employed.

### 8.8.3 Vacuum Crystallizers

Vacuum crystallizers produce supersaturated conditions by solvent removal and cooling [Figure 8.6(c)]. A hot concentrated solution is fed to an agitated crystallization chamber maintained at low pressure. The solution boils and cools adiabatically to the boiling point corresponding to the operating pressure. Crystallization follows concentration, and the product is removed from the bottom of the vessel. The principles of Oslo crystallizers are also employed in vacuum crystallization.

# 9

# Evaporation and Distillation

## 9.1 EVAPORATION

Evaporation may be defined as the removal of a solvent from a solution by vaporization, but is usually restricted to the concentration of solutions by boiling. Crystallization and drying, which may also utilize the vaporization of a liquid, are considered in subsequent sections. In the pharmaceutical industry evaporation is primarily associated with removing, by boiling, water and other solvents in batch processes. However, the principles governing such processes apply more generally and are derived from studying heat transfer to the boiling liquid, the relevant physical properties of the liquid, and the thermal stability of its components.

## 9.2 HEAT TRANSFER TO BOILING LIQUIDS IN AN EVAPORATOR

The heat required to boil a liquid in an evaporator is usually transferred from a heating fluid, such as steam or hot water, across the wall of a jacket or tube in or around which the liquid boils. A qualitative discussion of the methods used to secure high rates of heat flow can be based on equation 2.9:

$$Q = UA\Delta T \tag{2.9}$$

where $Q$ is the rate of heat flow, $U$ is the overall heat transfer coefficient, $A$ is the area over which heat is transferred, and $\Delta T$ is the difference in temperature between the fluids.

The overall heat transfer coefficient is derived from a series of individual coefficients that characterize the thermal barriers opposing heat transfer. Thus, for the heating fluid, the film coefficient for a condensing vapor, such as steam, is high provided that permanent gases and condensate are removed by venting and draining. With liquid heating media, the velocity of flow over the heat transfer surface should be as high as is practicable. If the solid barrier consists of a thin metal wall, the resistance to heat flow is small. Resistance, however, is significantly increased by chemical scale which may be deposited on either side. The accumulation of scale should be prevented. A glass wall may provide the largest thermal resistance of the system. Neglecting the thermal stability of the boiling liquid, circulation of the liquid should be rapid and, because of its influence on viscosity, the temperature of boiling should be as high as possible. Both factors promote high film coefficients on the product side of the wall.

Other factors described by equation 2.9 are the area of the heat transfer surfaces, which should be as large as possible, and the temperature difference between the heating surface and the boiling liquid. As long as the critical heat flux is not exceeded, the latter should also be large.

## 9.3 PHYSICAL PROPERTIES OF SOLUTION AND LIQUIDS

A number of physical factors, which are interrelated in a complex way, are relevant to a study of evaporation. For a given heating fluid the temperature difference across the wall of an evaporator is determined by the boiling temperature, a variable controlled by the external pressure and the solute concentration in the solution. The boiling temperature and the solute concentration influence the viscosity of the solution, a factor which greatly affects the heat transfer coefficient. The boiling temperature also determines the solubility of dissolved constituents and the degree of concentration which can be carried out without separation of solids.

### 9.3.1 Relation Between Boiling Temperature and Solute Concentration

When a solute is dissolved in a solvent, the vapor pressure is depressed and the boiling point rises. Since the boiling point increases as the solute concentration increases, the temperature difference between the boiling liquid and the heating surface falls. For dilute solutions the expected rise in boiling point can be calculated from Raoult's law. However, this procedure is not applicable to concentrated solutions or to solutions of uncertain composition. For aqueous concentrated solutions, Duhring's rule may be used to obtain the boiling point rise of a solution at any pressure. This rule states that the boiling point of a given solution is a linear function of the boiling point of water at the same pressure. A family of lines is required to cover a range of concentration as shown in Figure 9.1.

### 9.3.2 Relation of Boiling Temperature and External Pressure

The temperature at which a solution of given composition boils is determined by the external pressure. The vapor pressure of a pure solvent at any temperature can usually be obtained from published tables. Alternatively, if the vapor

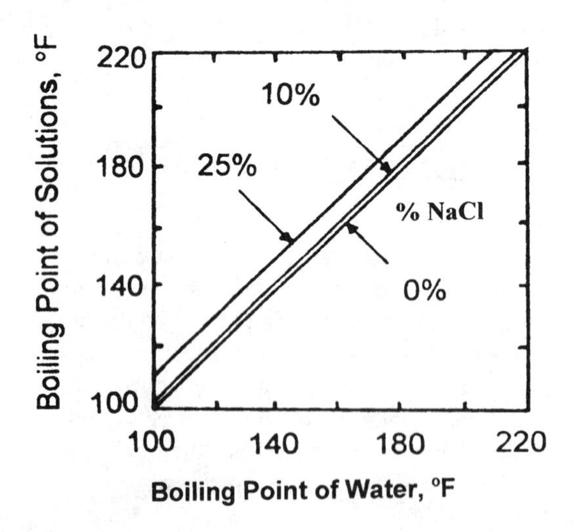


**FIGURE 9.1** Duhring chart for sodium chloride.

pressure at two temperatures is known, the plot of the logarithm of the vapor pressure against the reciprocal of the absolute temperature yields an approximately straight line. For intermediate pressures the temperature at which the solvent boils can be found by interpolation. If dissolved substances are present, the boiling point must be adjusted by using Duhring's rule. This value permits an accurate estimate of the temperature differences in the evaporator.

Reduction in the external pressure lowers the boiling temperature and, if the associated increase in viscosity is not too great, increases the rate of evaporation. On large installations a moderate vacuum is widely used to increase evaporator capacity. The imposition of low pressures and low boiling temperatures is also necessary when thermolabile materials are processed.

Boiling in tubes is commonly used in evaporators. In these circumstances the hydrostatic head developed by a column of liquid or the friction head imposed by its movement can create a local increase in pressure which suppresses boiling and decreases the evaporating capacity of the system.

### 9.3.3 Relation of Viscosity to Temperature and Solute Concentration

The viscosity of a solution is modified by changes in temperature and solute concentration. Since a low viscosity promotes a high heat transfer coefficient, the exponential decrease of viscosity with increase in temperature is of great importance and indicates a high boiling temperature.

In general, adding a nonvolatile solute increases a solution's viscosity at any temperature. Consequently, the viscosity increases as evaporation proceeds. These effects, however, cannot be calculated.

If at the operating temperatures and concentrations the viscosity of a solution is high, satisfactory heat transfer coefficients may only be obtained if the liquid is driven over the heating surface. In other systems, movement of a viscous liquid is assisted by gravity, or the liquid in contact with the heating surface is disrupted mechanically by scrapers.

### 9.3.4 Effect of Temperature on Solubility

The solubility of a solution's components depends on temperature. Most commonly, solubility increases with increase in temperature, so a greater degree of concentration is possible at higher temperatures without the separation of solids. The reverse is true of liquids containing scale-forming solids with inverse solubility characteristics, such as calcium or magnesium sulfate, or materials which decompose and deposit, such as coagulable protein.

### 9.3.5 Effect of Heat on the Active Constituents of a Solution

The thermal stability of components of a solution may determine the type of evaporator to be used and the conditions of its operation. If a simple solution contains a hydrolyzable material and the rate of its degradation during evaporation depends on its concentration at any time, an exponential relation between the remaining fraction, $F$, and the time, $t$, characteristic of a first-order reaction, is obtained:

$$F = e^{-kt} \tag{9.1}$$

The dependence of the reaction velocity constant, $k$, on the absolute temperature, $T$, is expressed by the relation

$$k = Ae^{-B/T} \tag{9.2}$$

where $A$ and $B$ are constants characteristic of the reaction. Thus, at temperatures $T_1$, $T_2$, and $T_3$, where $T_1 > T_2 > T_3$, the relation between remaining fraction and time of heating shown in Figure 9.2 emerges. This indicates the importance of the temperature and time of heating. If the latter can be shortened, the evaporation temperature can be greatly increased without increasing the

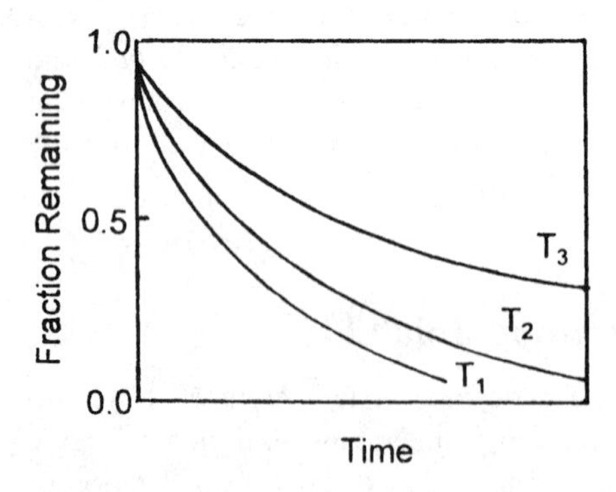


**FIGURE 9.2** Effect of time and temperature on degradation.

fraction which is degraded. If, therefore, the effect of temperature on evaporation rate is known, it is possible to define conditions of time and temperature at which decomposition is a minimum.

In practice, the kinetics of degradation and the relation of evaporation rate and temperature are usually not known, particularly when the criteria by which the product is judged are color, taste, or smell. In addition, this analysis neglects temperature variation in the evaporating liquid and degradation in boundary films where temperatures are higher. Often, therefore, experiments are necessary to determine the suitability of an evaporation process.

In batch processes the time of exposure to heat is well defined. This is also true of continuous processes in which the liquid to be evaporated is passed only once through the heater. In continuous processes in which the liquid is recirculated through the heater, the average residence time, $a$, given by the ratio (working volume of evaporator)/(volumetric discharge), in which volumetric discharge is only an indication of the damage which prolonged heating may cause. If perfect mixing occurs in the evaporator, the fraction, $f$, which is in the unit for time, $t$, or less is given by

$$f = 1 - e^{-t/a} \tag{9.3}$$

This relation shows, for example, that an evaporator with an average residence time of 1 hr holds 13.5% of active principles for 2 hr and about 2% for 4 hr.

## 9.4 EVAPORATORS

It is convenient to classify evaporators into the following: natural circulation evaporators, forced circulation evaporators, and film evaporators.

### 9.4.1 Natural Circulation Evaporators

Small-scale evaporators consist of a simple pan heated by a jacket, a coil, or by both. Admission of the heating fluid to the jacket induces a pool boiling regime in the vessel. Very small evaporators may be open, the vapor escaping to the atmosphere or into a vented hood. Larger pan evaporators are closed, the vapor being led away by pipe. Small jacketed pans are efficient, easy to clean, and may be fitted for the vacuum evaporation of thermolabile materials. However, because the ratio of heating area to volume decreases as the capacity increases, their size is limited and larger vessels must employ a heating coil. This improves evaporating capacity but makes cleaning more difficult.

The large heating area of a tube bundle is utilized widely in large-scale evaporators. Horizontal mounting, with the heating fluid inside the tube, is limited by poor circulation to the evaporation of nonviscous liquids in which the bundle is immersed. Normally, the tube bundle is mounted vertically and is known as a *calandria*. The boiling of liquids in a vertical tube and the earlier regimes of this process operate in a calandria. The tube lengths and the liquid level are such that boiling occurs in the tubes and the mixture of vapor and liquid rises until the entire calandria is just submerged. A typical evaporator is shown in Figure 9.3(a). The tubes are from 120 to 180 cm long and 5.1 to 7.6 cm in diameter. The low density of the boiling liquid and vapor creates an upward movement in the tubes. Vapor and liquid separate in the space above the calandria, and the liquid is returned to the pool at the base of the tubes by a large central downcomer or through an annular space between the heating element and the evaporator shell. Feed is added and concentrate is withdrawn from the pool as shown in the figure. As long as the liquid viscosity is low, good circulation and high heat transfer coefficients are obtained.

In some evaporators, the calandria is inclined and the tubes are lengthened.

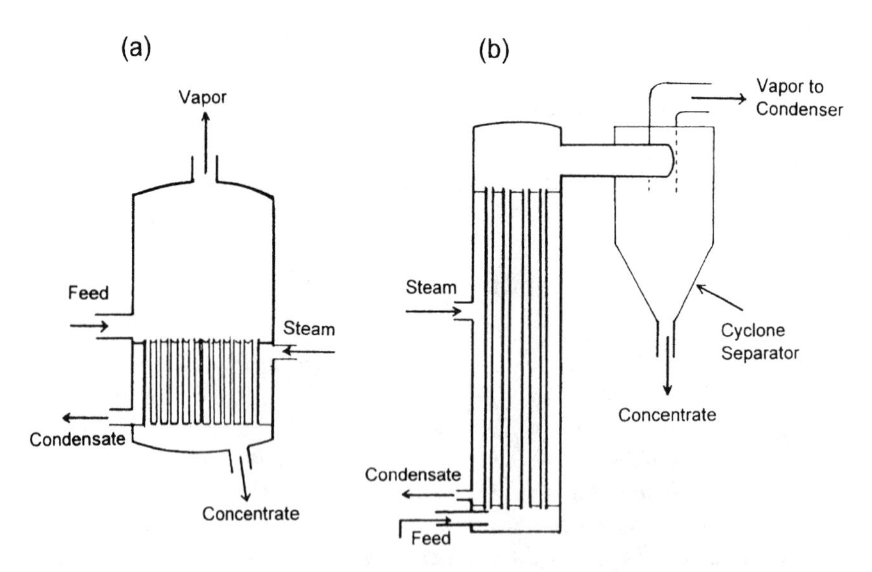


**FIGURE 9.3** (a) Evaporator with calandria and (b) climbing film evaporator.

## 9.4.2 Forced Circulation Evaporators

On the smallest scale, forced circulation evaporators are similar to pan evaporators, modified only by the inclusion of an agitator. Vigorous agitation increases the boiling film coefficient, the degree depending on the type and speed of the agitator. When evaporating viscous materials, one should use an agitator to prevent material degradation at the heated surfaces.

Some large-scale continuous units are similar to natural circulation evaporators. The natural circulation induced by boiling in a vertical tube may be supplemented by an axial impeller mounted in the downcomer of the calandria. This modification is used when viscous liquids or liquids containing suspended solids are evaporated. Such units are employed in evaporative crystallization. In other forced circulation evaporators, the tube bundle becomes, in effect, a simple heat exchanger, through the tubes of which the liquid is pumped. Commonly, the opposing head suppresses boiling in the tubes. Superheating occurs and the liquid flashes into a mixture of liquid and vapor as it enters the evaporator body.

## 9.4.3 Film Evaporators

In the calandria's short tubes an intimate mixture of vapor and liquid is discharged at the top. If the tube length is greatly increased, progressive phase separation occurs until a high-velocity core of vapor is formed, which propels an annular film of liquid along the tube. This phenomenon, which is one stage of flow when a liquid and a gas pass in the same direction along a tube, is employed in film evaporators. The turbulence of the film gives very high heat transfer coefficients, and the bubbles and vapor evolved are rapidly swept into the vapor stream. Although recirculation may be adopted, it is possible, with the high evaporation rates found in long tubes, to concentrate the liquid sufficiently in a single pass. Since a very short residence time is obtained, highly thermolabile materials may be concentrated at relatively high temperatures. Film evaporators are also suitable for materials which foam badly. Various types have been developed, but all are essentially continuous in operation, their capacity ranging from a few gallons per hour upward.

The climbing film evaporator, which is the most common film evaporator, consists of tubes 460 to 910 cm long and 2.5 to 5.1 cm in diameter mounted in a steam chest [Figure 9.3(b)]. The feed liquid enters the bottom of the tubes and flows upward for a short distance before boiling begins. The length of this section, which is characterized by low-heat-transfer coefficients, may be minimized by preheating the feed to its boiling point. The pattern of boiling and phase separation follows, and a mixture of liquid and vapor emerges from the top of the tube to be separated by baffles or by a cyclone separator. Climbing film evaporators are not suitable for evaporating viscous liquids.

In the falling film evaporator the liquid is fed to the top of long heated tubes. Since gravity assists flow down the tube, this arrangement is better suited to the evaporation of moderately viscous liquids. The vapor evolved is usually carried downward, and the mixture of liquid and vapor emerges from the bottom for separation. Even distribution of liquid must be secured during feeding. A tendency to channel in some tubes leads to drying in others.

The rising-falling film evaporator concentrates a liquid in a climbing film section and then leads the emerging liquid and vapor into a second tube section which forms a falling film evaporator. Good distribution in the falling film section is claimed, and the evaporator is particularly suitable for liquids which increase greatly in viscosity during evaporation.

In mechanically aided film evaporators a thin film of material is maintained on the heat transfer surface irrespective of the viscosity. This is usually achieved by a rotor, concentric with the tube, which carries blades that scrape the tube or ride with low clearance in the film. Mechanical agitation permits evaporation of materials which are highly viscous or have a low thermal conductivity. Since temperature variations in the film are reduced and residence times are shortened, the vacuum evaporation of viscous thermolabile materials becomes possible.

### 9.4.4 Efficiency of Evaporators

In the pharmaceutical industry economic use of steam may not be of overriding importance because the small scale of the operation and the high value of the product do not justify the additional capital costs of improved heating efficiency. In other industries heating costs require more efficient use of heat. This efficiency is secured by utilizing the heat content of the vapor emerging from the evaporator, assumed, until now, to be lost in a following condensation. Two methods commonly used are multiple-effect evaporation and vapor recompression.

In multiple-effect evaporation, the vapor from one evaporator is led as the heating medium to the calandria of a second evaporator, which, therefore, must operate at a lower temperature than the first. This principle can be extended to a number of evaporators, some stages working under vacuum. The limit is set by the relation of the cost of the plant and the vacuum services to the cost of the steam saved.

In evaporators employing vapor recompression, the vapor emerging is compressed by mechanical pumps or steam jet ejectors to increase its temperature. The compressed vapor is returned to the steam chest.

### 9.4.5 Vapor Removal and Liquid Entrainment

Vapor must be removed from the evaporator with as little entrained liquid as possible. The two determining factors are the vapor velocity at the surface of the liquid and the velocity of the vapor leaving the evaporator. On a small scale, surface vapor velocities will be low but with increase in scale, the adverse ratio of surface area to volume creates higher velocities. Droplets formed by the bubbles bursting at the boiling surface may then be projected from the surface. In addition, foam may form. Various devices may be used to control entrainment at or near the surface. A high vapor space is provided above the boiling liquid to allow large droplets to fall and foam to collapse. Baffles may be used in the vapor space to arrest entrained droplets. Where allowable, antifoaming agents, such as silicone oils, can be used to depress foaming.

Stokes' law shows that vapor of particular characteristics will carry droplets upward against the force of gravity. Any entrained liquid not intercepted in the evaporator body is, therefore, carried forward in the higher-velocity stream of the vapor uptake. Some droplets are caught here, the quantity depending on duct geometry and vapor velocity. At atmospheric pressure, the latter might be 17 m $s^{-1}$. In vacuum evaporation much higher velocities may be used. When the quantity of entrained liquid is high, the vapor is commonly led to a cyclone separator, which is used with frothing materials, and to the vapor-liquid mixture leaving a climbing film evaporator. In the separator the entrained liquid is flung out to the walls by centrifugal force and may be collected or returned to the evaporator. The vapor is led to a condenser.

### 9.4.6 Evaporation Without Boiling

During heating, some evaporation takes place at the surface of a batch of liquid before boiling begins. Similarly, liquids which are very viscous or which froth excessively may be concentrated without boiling. The diffusion of vapor from the surface is then described by equation 3.5:

$$N_A = \frac{k_g}{RT}(P_{Ai} - P_{Ag}) \tag{3.5}$$

where $N_A$ is the number of moles evaporating from unit area in unit time, $k_g$ is the mass transfer coefficient (proportional to the gas velocity) across the boundary layer, $R$ is the gas constant, $T$ is the absolute temperature, $P_{Ai}$ is the liquid vapor pressure, and $P_{Ag}$ is the partial pressure of the vapor in the gas stream.

## 9.5 DISTILLATION

Distillation is a process in which a liquid mixture is separated into its component parts by vaporization. The vapor evolved from a boiling liquid mixture is normally richer in the more volatile components than the liquid with which it is in equilibrium. Distillation rests upon this fact. Although multicomponent mixtures are most common in distillation processes, an understanding of the operation can be based on the vapor pressure characteristics of two component or binary mixtures. Binary systems in which the liquids are immiscible are discussed first. Discussion of the separation of miscible liquids by fractionation forms most of the remainder of the section.

## 9.6 BINARY MIXTURES OF IMMISCIBLE LIQUIDS: STEAM DISTILLATION

If the two components of a binary mixture are immiscible, the vapor pressure of the mixture is the sum of the vapor pressures of the two components, each exerted independently and not as a function of their relative concentrations in the liquid. This property is employed in steam distillation, a process particularly applicable to the separation of high-boiling-point substances from non-volatile impurities. The steam forms a cheap and inert carrier. The principles of the process, however, apply to other immiscible systems.

If a mixture of water and a high-boiling liquid, such as nitrobenzene, is heated, the total vapor pressure increases and ultimately reaches the external pressure. The mixture boils and the vapors evolved are condensed to give a liquid mixture which separates under gravity. In practice, the vapors are produced by blowing steam into the liquid in a manner which gives intimate contact between the phases. Since both components contribute to the total pressure, the boiling temperature must be lower than the boiling point of either component. In the case of nitrobenzene and water, the boiling point at atmospheric pressure is about 372 K. To distill nitrobenzene alone at this temperature, a pressure of 20 mm Hg must be imposed. Steam distillation, therefore, permits the distillation of water-immiscible materials of high boiling point without the use of high temperatures, which might cause decomposition, or high vacua. The method, however, only separates such materials from nonvolatile constituents. If volatile impurities are present, they appear in the distillate.

The composition of the distillate is calculated in the following way. For two components, A and B, the total vapor pressure, $P$, is the sum of the vapor pressures of the components, $P_A$ and $P_B$. Since the partial pressure of a component in a gaseous mixture is proportional to its molar concentration, the vapor composition is

$$\frac{n_A}{n_B} = \frac{P_A}{P_B} \tag{9.4}$$

where $n_A$ and $n_B$ are the number of moles of A and B in the vapor, respectively. If $W_A$ and $W_B$ are the weights of A and B in the vapor, then

$$\frac{W_A}{M_A}\frac{M_B}{W_B} = \frac{P_A}{P_B} \tag{9.5}$$

where $M_A$ and $M_B$ are the respective molecular weights. The distillate obtained from the vapor is $W_A + W_B$. Therefore,

$$\text{Percentage of A in distillate} = \frac{W_A}{W_A + W_B} \times 100 = \frac{P_A M_A}{P_A M_A + P_B M_B} \times 100 \tag{9.6}$$

The ratio of immiscible organic liquid to water in the distillate is increased if the former has a high molecular weight or a high vapor pressure.

Steam distillation under vacuum may be employed when the thermal stability of the material prohibits temperatures of about 373 K. A further variant is the introduction of unsaturated steam under conditions in which no condensation to water takes place. Only two phases, the liquid being distilled and the mixed vapors, are then present. The external pressure no longer fixes the temperature, as in a three-phase system, and any convenient value can be chosen.

The chief uses of steam distillation are the purification and isolation of liquids of high boiling point, such as aniline, nitrobenzene, or σ-dichlorobenzene, and in the preparation of fatty acids and volatile oils. Many of the latter are prepared by introducing steam into a mixture of the comminuted drug and water. The method is also used to remove odoriferous elements, such as aldehydes and ketones, from edible oils. Dehydrating a material by adding a volatile water-immiscible solvent, such as toluene, and distilling the mixture is a form of steam distillation. The solvent separates in the condensate and may be returned to the still.

## 9.7 BINARY MIXTURES OF MISCIBLE LIQUIDS

### 9.7.1 Relation of Vapor Pressure and Mixture Composition

When the two components of a binary mixture are completely miscible, the vapor pressure of a mixture is a function of mixture composition as well as the vapor pressures of the two pure components. If the liquids are ideal, the relationship of vapor pressure and composition is given by Raoult's law. At constant temperature the partial vapor pressure of a constituent of an ideal mixture is proportional to its mole fraction in the liquid. Thus, for a mixture of A and B,

$$P_A = P_A^\circ x_A \tag{9.7}$$

where $P_A$ is the partial vapor pressure of A in the mixture, $P_A^\circ$ is the vapor pressure of pure A, and $x_A$ is its mole fraction. Similarly,

$$P_B = P_B^\circ x_B \tag{9.8}$$

The total pressure of the system, $P$, is simply $P_A + P_B$.

These relations can be expressed graphically. If the vapor pressure at a given temperature of each pure component is marked on a graph of vapor pressure versus mole fraction, the total vapor pressure at the same temperature of a liquid mixture of any composition falls on the straight line joining the vapor pressures of the two components. The partial pressure of each component is indicated by the diagonals of this figure. The principle is shown in Figure 9.4. A separate relation must be constructed for each temperature.

Very few liquid mixtures rigidly obey Raoult's law. Consequently, the vapor pressure data must be determined experimentally. Mixtures which deviate positively from the law give a total vapor pressure curve that lies above the theoretical straight line. Negative deviations fall below the line. In extreme cases deviations are so large that a range of mixtures exhibits a vapor pressure higher or lower than either of the pure components.

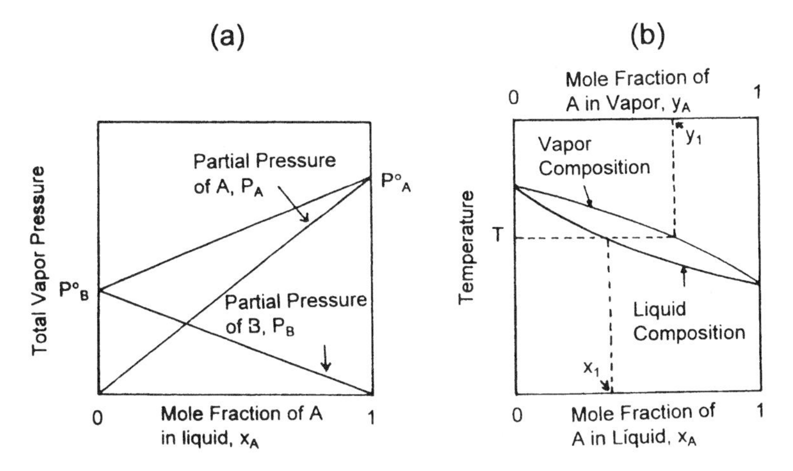


**FIGURE 9.4** (a) Vapor pressure of an ideal binary mixture; (b) phase diagram.

Returning to ideal systems, the partial pressure of a component in the vapor is proportional to its mole fraction. For component A,

$$P_A = y_A P \tag{9.9}$$

where $P_A$ is the partial pressure of A in the vapor and $y_A$ is its mole fraction. Since $P_A = P_A^{\circ} x_A$,

$$y_A = \frac{x_A \, P_B^{\circ}}{P} \tag{9.10}$$

Similarly,

$$y_B = \frac{x_B P_B^{\circ}}{P} \tag{9.11}$$

If A is the more volatile component, $P_A^{\circ} > P$; therefore, $y_A > x_A$; i.e., the vapor is richer in the more volatile component than the liquid with which it is in equilibrium.

## 9.7.2 The Relation of Boiling Point and Mixture Composition

For the purposes of distillation, curves relating vapor pressure and composition are usually replaced by boiling point curves. These are determined by experi-

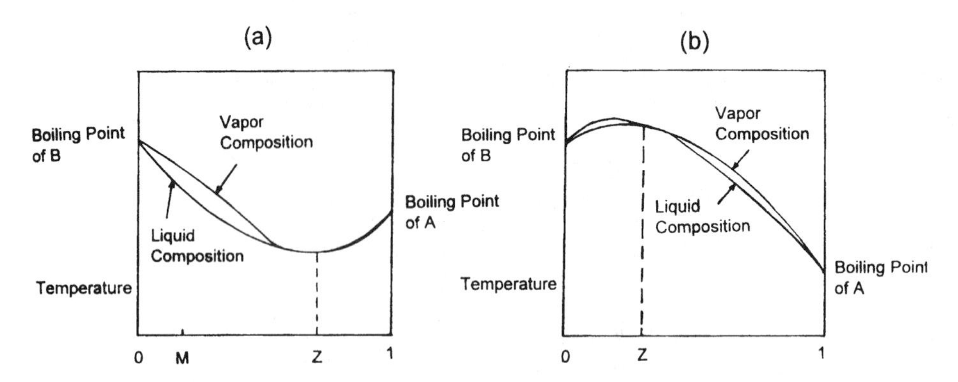


**FIGURE 9.5** Temperature-composition diagrams for a binary mixture: (a) minimum azeotrope; (b) maximum azeotrope.

ment at the given pressure. Figure 9.5(a) represents a system in which the vapor pressure of some mixtures is greater than the vapor pressure of the pure, more volatile component. This system exhibits a minimum boiling point, and the composition of the liquid at this point is *Z*. This mixture, which is a constant boiling or azeotropic mixture, evolves on boiling a vapor of the same composition. In the binary system described in Figure 9.5(b), mixtures are formed with a vapor pressure less than that of the less volatile component. The maximum boiling point is given by the azeotropic mixture, *Z*.

Systems forming minimum boiling mixtures are common, one example being ethyl alcohol and water, where, the azeotrope contains 4.5% by weight of water. The boiling point at atmospheric pressure is 351.15 K, 0.25 K lower than the boiling point of pure alcohol. Maximum boiling mixtures are less common. The most familiar example is hydrochloric acid, which forms an azeotrope boiling at 381 K and containing 20.2% by weight of hydrochloric acid.

Mixtures forming azeotropes cannot be separated into the pure components by normal distillation methods. However, separation into the azeotrope and one pure component is possible. Efficient fractionation of the mixture *M* of Figure 9.5(a) gives the azeotrope *Z* as distillate and pure B as the residue.

The composition of the azeotropic mixture of a system is a function of the total pressure, and it is possible in some cases to eliminate the constant boiling mixture by altering the pressure at which the distillation is performed. For example, at pressures less than 100 mm Hg, ethyl alcohol and water do not form an azeotrope, and can be completely separated.

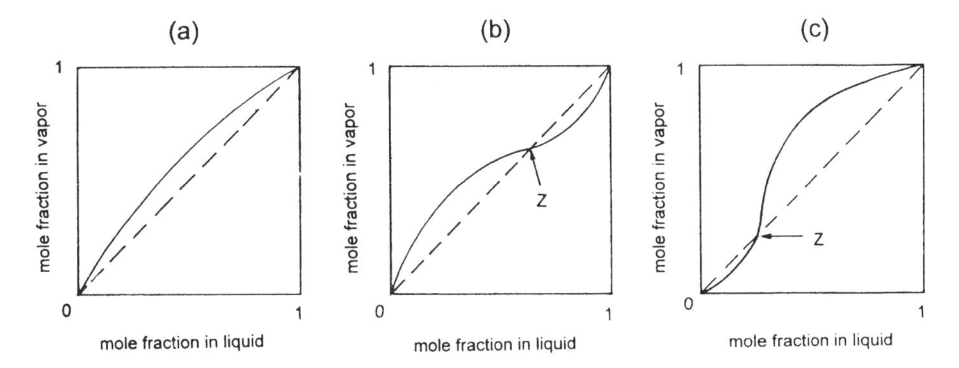


**FIGURE 9.6** Vapor-liquid equilibrium diagrams.

### 9.7.3 Vapor-Liquid Equilibrium Diagrams

Vapor-liquid equilibrium diagrams (Figure 9.6) are an alternative and convenient method of recording distillation data. They consist of a conventional graph relating the mole fraction of the more volatile component in the liquid, $X$, to the mole fraction of the more volatile component in the vapor, $Y$. An ideal binary system is shown in Figure 9.6(a). The temperature varies along each of the curves, and the diagram is only applicable to the pressure at which the variables were measured. Curves of minimum boiling mixtures and maximum boiling mixtures are drawn in Figure 9.6(b) and Figure 9.6(c), respectively.

## 9.8 SIMPLE OR DIFFERENTIAL DISTILLATION

In simple or differential distillation, the vapor evolved from the boiling mixture is immediately removed and condensed. For the system in Figure 9.7(a), the liquid of composition $x_1$ evolves a vapor of composition $y_1$. Its removal impoverishes the liquid in the more volatile component. The composition of the liquid moves toward pure B and its boiling point increases. There is, therefore, a progressive change in the vapor composition, the mole fraction of the more volatile component steadily decreasing. Unless the boiling points of the two pure components differ widely, a reasonable degree of separation is not possible. The method may be used to remove low-boiling-point solvents from aqueous solutions.

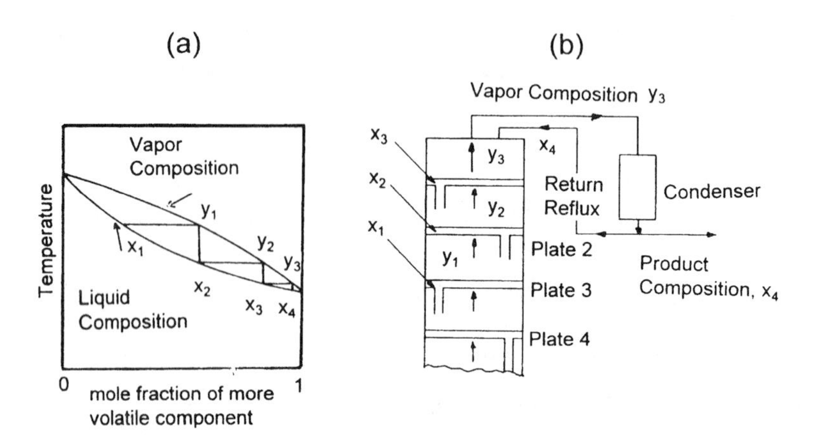


**FIGURE 9.7** (a) Three ideal stages in a fractional distillation and (b) the plate column associated with the fractional distillation.

## 9.9 RECTIFICATION OR FRACTIONATION

In simple distillation, vapor enrichment is small. In fractionation, a term synonymous with rectification, the vapor leaving the boiling liquid is led up a column to meet a liquid stream or reflux which originates higher in the column as part of the condensate. In a series of partial condensations and vaporizations, the rising vapor becomes richer in the more volatile component at the expense of the falling liquid, and high degrees of separation are possible. The columns, called *fractionating columns*, are of two basic types: packed columns and plate columns.

Packed columns are used for laboratory and small-scale industrial distillation and are usually operated as a batch process. The column consists of a vertical, hollow, cylindrical shell containing a packing designed to offer a large interfacial contact area between liquid and vapor. The form of the packing varies, but Raschig rings, which consist of small metallic or ceramic cylinders, are the most commonly used. Other shapes are saddles, Pall rings, Lessing rings, and meshes of woven wire or expanded metal. In a packed column, countercurrent interaction between the rising vapor and the falling liquid occurs throughout the column length. The distillation rate and the size and shape of the packing must be chosen to give efficient support for the liquid phase, phase movement, and phase interaction. High rates of vapor flow may arrest or reverse the downward movement of liquid. This ultimately causes column flooding and determines the upper end of the operating range. The column efficiency is also decreased if the falling liquid fails to wet all the available packing surface, a condition which determines the lower limit of column operation. In general, packed columns operate under widely varying conditions without serious loss of efficiency.

### 9.9.1 Plate Columns

A plate column consists of a series of plates or trays on which the liquid is retained for some period during its movement down the column. The rising vapor is bubbled through this liquid, providing intimate contact between the phases. Liquid in reflux moves downward between plates and is usually carried by a downcomer. Contact between the vapor and liquid takes place in stages. Plate columns operate efficiently over a limited range of conditions. They are mainly used in large-scale, continuous installations in which the conditions of distillation can be closely maintained.

### 9.9.2 Principles of Continuous and Batch Fractionation

Figure 9.7(a) is the boiling point curve of a binary mixture. If a mixture of composition $x_1$ is boiled, a vapor of composition $y_1$ is evolved, and condensation gives a liquid of composition $x_2$. This is an ideal distillation stage. A second stage gives a liquid of composition $x_3$, and, in this example, a further stage would give the more volatile component in an almost pure form.

These conditions are approached in continuously operated fractionating columns. In such columns, operating with continuous feed and product withdrawal, the composition of the liquid and vapor at any point does not vary with time. The process is examined with reference to the plate column in Figure 9.7(b). Let the composition of the liquid on plate 3 be $x_1$. The vapor received at this plate from the plate below is bubbled through the liquid on the plate. Some of the less volatile component is condensed, increasing the mole fraction of the more volatile component in the bubbles. The latent heat evolved by this condensation vaporizes some of the liquid on the plate. This vapor is richer in the more volatile component than the liquid is. By these two mechanisms the vapor which will leave the plate moves toward equilibrium with the liquid on the plate. If equilibrium could be achieved, maximum enrichment of the vapor would occur corresponding to the appropriate horizontal line linking vapor-liquid equilibrium concentrations on the boiling point curve. For the system in Figure 9.7(b), this line is $x_1y_1$. Two more ideal distillation stages at plates 2 and 1 complete the separation of this mixture. In practice, equilibrium is not achieved at the plates due to limited contact between the phases. Enrichment is therefore less than that at an ideal stage and the discrepancy is a measure of plate efficiency.

Under steady column conditions, the concentration of the more volatile component in the liquid on any plate is maintained by the overflow or reflux of liquid richer in the more volatile component from the plate above. This is true of all parts except the top plate. Here, the mole fraction of the more volatile component must be maintained by returning part of the condensate from the last stage to the top plate. This is known as reflux return, and the reflux ratio is the ratio of the condensate returned to the column and the amount withdrawn as product. This ratio markedly affects the degree of separation occurring in a given column. If the proportion of the condensate to be returned to the column is increased, the mole fraction of the more volatile component in the liquid on the top plate is increased. The mole fraction of this component in the emerging vapor is also increased and a purer product is obtained. By the increased overflow of liquid from plate to plate down the column, this is also true of all plates. Thus, by increasing the reflux ratio, the enrichment obtained with a given number of plates is increased. The amount of product, however, is decreased. A column operating at total reflux, in which the whole of the distillate is returned to the column, achieves a given enrichment with a minimum number of plates. This column, however, gives no product at all, and an economic compromise is sought between a short column with a small number of plates operating with high reflux ratio and a long column of many plates operating with a low reflux ratio.

Algebraic and graphical methods are used to calculate the theoretical number of plates required to separate a mixture in a column operating with a known reflux ratio. In a packed column, enrichment of the vapor takes place continuously as the column is ascended. The enrichment taking place over a certain length of the column corresponds to the enrichment secured at a plate which behaves ideally. This correspondence is expressed as the height equivalent of a theoretical or ideal plate (HETP). This concept allows the account given for plate columns to be directly applied to packed columns. The packing height required for a separation is simply the product of the HETP and the number of ideal stages required. The HETP is not constant for a given packing, but depends on the physical properties of the liquid and the vapor, such as density and viscosity, and on the distillation rate.

In batch distillation, steady-state conditions are never achieved, and the concentration of the more volatile component in the still or at any point in the column falls as the rich product is withdrawn from the top. The concentration of the more volatile component in the product also falls. To maintain a given product specification, it may be necessary to increase the reflux ratio from time to time. Alternatively, the reflux ratio could be so chosen that the average composition of the product complies with the specification, the first distillate being enriched and the last depleted of the more volatile component.

Most distillations, whether operated as batch or continuous processes, are applied to mixtures of more than two components. If the boiling points of the components differ widely, the process may be treated as successive distillation of two component mixtures. If a mixture of three components, A, B, and C, is batch-distilled, a column with sufficient plates will initially separate the most volatile component, A, with a high purity. As distillation progresses, the concentration of A in the distillate falls, and, ultimately, the column fails to produce a distillate of the required quality. An intermediate fraction is then distilled, consisting of A and B, until the distillate contains the required amount of B. After this fraction is collected, a second intermediate fraction is distilled to leave component C in the still. Intermediate fractions can be distilled with subsequent batches. A similar separation could be accomplished with two continuous columns, one separating A from B and C and another separating B from C.

To avoid thermal decomposition of a component in a mixture, distillation may be performed at a reduced pressure. In addition to the general principles we have described, the following factors may be important. The pressure drop associated with the flow of vapor up the column, which is relatively small in atmospheric distillation, may become significant, producing a damaging increase in the temperature of the liquid in the still. Second, in packed columns, flooding occurs at lower distillation rates due to the high velocity of the rising vapor.

## 9.10 SEPARATION OF AZEOTROPES AND LIQUIDS OF SIMILAR VOLATILITY

Systems which form azeotropes cannot be separated by fractional distillation, although formation of the azeotrope can sometimes be precluded by changing the distillation pressure. Problems of separation are also found with mixtures of liquids with similar volatility. Separation of these systems can be facilitated by adding a third component. If this component forms one or more azeotropes with the original components of the mixture, the process is called *azeotropic distillation*. The addition of a relatively nonvolatile component which alters the relative volatility of the original components gives a process known as *extractive distillation*.

In azeotropic distillation of minimum-boiling binary mixtures, the third component either forms a new binary azeotrope of lower boiling point or a ternary azeotrope of lower boiling point containing the original components in different proportions. The newly formed azeotrope must be easily separated after distillation. The process is illustrated by the dehydration of alcohol with benzene. The binary azeotrope of ethyl alcohol and water boils at 351.15 K, the ternary azeotrope of benzene, water, and alcohol boils at 337.8 K, and the binary azeotrope of benzene and alcohol boils at 341 K. Distillation of the alcohol-water azeotrope with benzene yields the ternary azeotrope, which separates on condensation to give two layers, one of which contains almost all the water. In a batch process the column then gives the benzene alcohol azeotrope, leaving anhydrous alcohol in the still. In a continuous process the various stages are each performed on a different column.

Extractive distillation is illustrated in the separation of benzene and cyclohexane by phenol addition. The relative volatility of the original components is modified so that cyclohexane is recovered as the distillate, leaving a mixture of phenol and benzene which is passed to a second column for separation. The phenol, which is added to the top of the column, appears to aid separation by preferentially dissolving benzene during its downward passage. This leads to the term *extractive distillation*.

## 9.11 MOLECULAR DISTILLATION

Molecular distillation is carried out without boiling at very low pressures, around 0.001 mmHg. At these pressures molecular collisions in the evolving vapor and their reflection back to the liquid surface are greatly decreased, and the mean free path of the molecules is of the same order as the distance between the evaporating surface and a condenser placed a short distance away. It then becomes possible to distill liquids of very high boiling point, although the degree of separation cannot exceed one theoretical plate. The process is therefore used primarily to concentrate nonvolatile components in a high-boiling-point medium. The vitamins in cod liver oil can be concentrated in this way. For separating liquids of comparable volatility several separate distillation stages are necessary.

Since agitation due to boiling is absent, an alternative method of maintaining the more volatile component at the evaporating surface must be

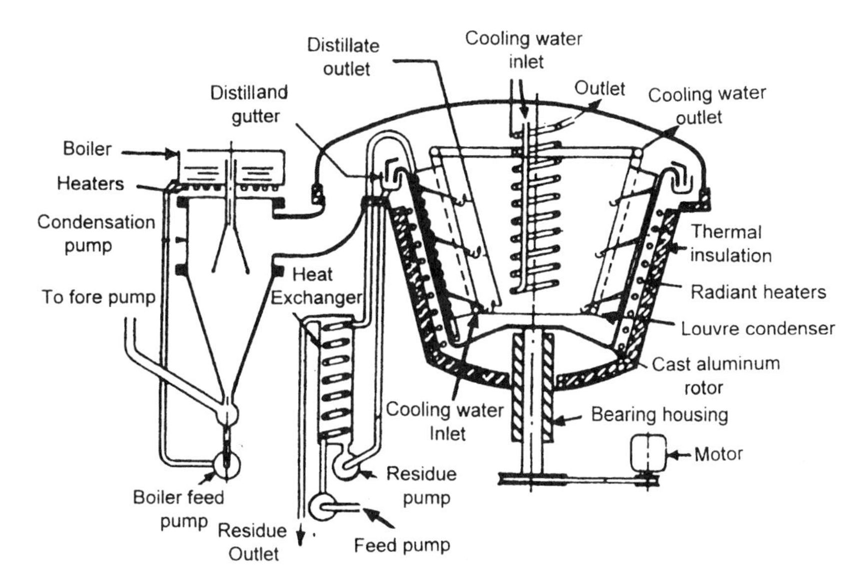


**FIGURE 9.8** Large-scale molecular still.

adopted. In the industrial molecular still in Figure 9.8, the feed is introduced at the bottom of a heated conical rotor and flows upward as a thin liquid layer under the action of centrifugal force. The residue is caught in a gutter at the top. The vapor is condensed on a concentric, water-cooled condenser a short distance away and discharged.

# 10

# Filtration

The student of pharmacy will have used filtration extensively in the collection of precipitates in chemical analyses or in the preparation of parenteral fluids and will, therefore, anticipate the definition of filtration as the removal of solids suspended in a liquid or gas by passage through a pervious medium on which the solids are retained. The pervious medium or septum is normally supported on a base, and these, together with a suitable housing providing free access of fluid to and from the septum, comprise the filter.

## 10.1 APPLICATIONS OF FILTRATION

The applications of filtration are diverse. They may, however, be classified as clarification or cake filtration.

### 10.1.1 Clarification

Very high standards of clarity are imposed during the production of pharmaceutical solutions. The aim may be simply the presentation of an elegant product, although complete freedom from particulate matter is obviously necessary in the manufacture of most parenteral solutions. The solids are unwanted and are normally present in a very small concentration. Clarification may be carried out by the use of thick media that allow for the penetration and arrest of particles by entrapment, impingement, and electrostatic effects. This leads to the concept of depth filtration in which particles, perhaps a hundred times smaller than the dimensions of the passages through the medium, are removed. For this reason, such filters are not absolute and must be designed with sufficient depth so that the probability of the passage of the smallest particle under consideration through the filter is extremely small.

Depth filtration differs fundamentally from the use of media in which pore size determines the size of particle retained. Such filters may be said to be ''absolute'' at a particle diameter closely related to the size of the pore, so there is a relatively sharp division between particles that pass the filter and those that are retained. An analogy with sieving may be drawn for this mechanism. The life of such filters depends on the number of available pores for fluid passage. Once a particle is trapped at the entrance to the pore, the pore's contribution to the overall flow of liquid is very much reduced. Coarse straining with a wire mesh and the membrane filter employ this mechanism.

Sterilization of liquids by filtration could be regarded as an extreme application of clarification in which the complete removal of particles as small as $0.3 \times 10^{-6}$ m must be ensured.

### 10.1.2 Cake Filtration

The most common industrial application is filtration of slurries containing a relatively large amount of suspended solids, usually 3% to 20%. The septum acts only as a support in this operation. The actual filtration is carried out by the solids deposited as a cake. In such cases, solids may completely penetrate the septum until the deposition of an effective cake occurs. Until this time, cloudy filtrate may be recycled. The physical properties of the cake largely determine the methods employed. Often, washing and partial drying or dewatering are integral parts of the process. Effective discharge of the cake completes the process. The solids, the filtrate, or both may be wanted.

## 10.2 FILTRATION THEORIES

Two aspects of filtration theory must be considered. The first describes the flow of fluids through porous media. It is applicable to both clarification and cake filtration. The second—which is of primary importance only in clarification—examines the retention of particles in a depth filter.

### 10.2.1 Fluid Flow Through Porous Media

The concept of a channel with a hydraulic diameter equivalent to the complex interstitial network that exists in a powder bed leads to the equation

$$Q = \frac{KA\ \Delta P}{\eta L} \tag{10.1}$$

where $Q$ is the volumetric flow rate, $A$ is the bed area, $L$ is the bed thickness, $\Delta P$ is the pressure difference across the bed, and $\eta$ is the fluid viscosity. The permeability coefficient, $K$, is

$$K = \frac{\varepsilon^3}{5(1 - \varepsilon)^2 S_0^2}$$

where $\varepsilon$ is the bed porosity and $S_0$ is the bed's specific surface area by volume ($m^2/m^3$).

### 10.2.2 Factors Affecting Filtration Rate

Equation 10.1 may be used as a basis for discussing those factors that determine the filtration rate.

#### Pressure

The filtration rate at any instant of time is directly proportional to the pressure difference across the bed. In cake filtration, deposition of solids over a finite period increases bed depth. If, therefore, the pressure remains constant, the filtration rate falls. Alternatively, the pressure can be progressively increased to maintain the filtration rate.

Conditions in which the pressure is substantially constant are found in vacuum filtration. In pressure filtration it is usual to employ a low constant pressure in the early stages of filtration, for reasons to be given. The pressure is then stepped up as the operation proceeds.

This analysis neglects the additional resistance derived from the supporting septum and the thin layer of particles associated with it. At the operation's beginning some particles penetrate the septum and are retained in the capillaries in the manner of depth filtration while other particles bridge the pores at the surface to begin the cake formation. The effect of penetration, which is analogous to blinding a sieve, is to confer a resistance on the cake-septum junction which is much higher than the resistance of the clean septum with a small associated layer of cake. This layer may contribute heavily to the total resistance. Since penetration is not reversible, the initial period of cake filtration is highly critical and is usually carried out at a low pressure. The amount of penetration depends on the septum structure, the size, shape, and concentration of the solid particles, and the filtration rate.

When clarifying at constant pressure, a slow decrease in filtration rate occurs because material is deposited within the bed.

## Viscosity

The inverse relation between flow rate and viscosity indicates that, as expected, higher pressures are required to maintain a given flow rate for thick liquids than are necessary for filtering thin liquids. The decrease in viscosity with increase in temperature may suggest the use of hot filtration. Some plants (e.g., the filter press) can be equipped so that the temperature of hot slurries can be maintained.

## Filter Area

In cake filtration a suitable filter area must be employed for a particular slurry. If this area is too small, the excessively thick cakes produced necessitate high-pressure differentials to maintain a reasonable flow rate. This is highly important in the filtration of slurries giving compressible cakes. When clarifying, the relation is simpler. The filtration rate can be doubled by simply doubling the filter area.

## Permeability Coefficient

The permeability coefficient may be examined in terms of its two variables: porosity and surface area: Evaluation of the term $\varepsilon^3/(1 - \varepsilon)^2$ shows that the permeability coefficient is a sensitive function of porosity. When a slurry is filtered, the cake porosity depends on the way in which particles are deposited and packed. A porosity or void fraction from 0.27 to 0.47 is possible in the regular arrangements of spheres of equal size. Intermediate values are normally obtained in the random deposition of deflocculated particles of fairly regular shape. A fast deposition rate, given by concentrated slurries or high flow rates, may give a higher porosity because of the greater possibility of bridging and arching in the cake. Although theoretically the particle size has no effect on porosity (assuming that the bed is large compared with the particles), a broad particle size distribution may lead to a reduction of porosity if small particles pack in the interstices created by larger particles.

Surface area, unlike porosity, is markedly affected by particle size and is inversely proportional to particle diameter. Hence, as commonly observed in the laboratory, a coarse precipitate is easier to filter than a fine precipitate even though both may pack with the same porosity. Where possible, a previous operation may be modified to facilitate filtration. For example, a suitable particle size may be obtained in a crystallization process by control of nucleation, or the proportion of fines in milling may be reduced by carefully controlling residence times. In most cases, however, control of this type is not possible, and, with materials that filter only with difficulty, much may be gained by conditioning the slurry, an operator that modifies the porosity and specific surface of the depositing cake.

In clarification, high permeability and filtration rate oppose good particle retention. In the formation of clarifying media from sintered or loose particles, accurate control of particle size, specific surface, and porosity is possible, so a medium can be designed that offers the best compromise between permeability and particle retention. This analysis of permeability can be accurately applied to these systems. Due to the extremes of shape, this is not so of the fibrous media used for clarification. Here it is possible to develop a material of high permeability and high retentive capacity. However, such a material is intrinsically weak and must be adequately supported.

### 10.2.3 Particle Retention in a Depth Filter

Theoretical studies of particle retention have been restricted to granular media of a type used in purifying municipal water. The aim is to predict the variation of filtrate quality with influent quality or time and then estimate the effect of removed solids on the permeability of the bed. Such studies have some bearing on the use of granular, sintered, or fibrous beds used for clarifying pharmaceuticals.

The path followed by the liquid through a bed is extremely tortuous. Violent changes of direction and velocity occur as the system of pores and waists is traversed. Deflection of particles by gravity or, for very fine particles, by Brownian movement brings particles within range of the attractive forces between particles and the medium and causes arrest. Inertial effects—that is, the movement of a particle across streamlines by virtue of its momentum—are considered to be important only when particles are removed from gases. In liquid-solid systems, density differences are much smaller.

Opportunity for contact and arrest depends on the surface area of the bed, the tortuosity of the void space, and the interstitial speed of the liquid.

Since the inertial mechanism is ineffective, increase in interstitial velocity decreases the opportunity for contact and retention of particles by the medium. Therefore, a filter's efficiency decreases as the flow rate increases. However, efficiency increases as the density or size of the influent particles increases and decreases as the particle size in the bed decreases. Each layer of clean filter is considered to remove the same proportion of particles in the influent. Mathematically expressed,

$$\frac{dC}{dx} = -KC \tag{10.2}$$

where $C$ is the concentration of particles entering element of depth $dx$. The value of $K$, which is a clarifying coefficient expressing the fraction of particles that deposit in unit depth of the bed, changes with time. Initially, the rate of removal increases and the efficiency of filtration improves, perhaps, as has been suggested, because the particle deposition in the bed is at first localized and the surface area and tortuosity increase. Later, the removal efficiency decreases because deposition narrows the pores, reduces convolutions and surface area, and increases the interstitial liquid velocity. The failure of the medium to adequately retain particles or the decrease in permeability and filtration rate eventually limit filter life. If deposition is reversible, then permeability and retentive capacity can be restored by vigorous backwashing. Alternatively, the medium should be cheap and expendable.

### 10.2.4 Conditioning of Slurries

The permeability of an ideal filter bed, such as that formed by a filter aid, is about $7 \times 10^{-13}$ m$^2$. This is more than 10,000 times the permeability of a precipitate of aluminum hydroxide. Therefore, modifying the slurry's physical properties, called *slurry conditioning*, can be a powerful tool for a filtration engineer. Two methods, flocculation and addition of filter aids, are discussed.

*Flocculation* of slurries is a common procedure in which the addition of flocculating agents is permissible. The aggregates or flocs, which are characterized by a high sedimentation rate and sedimentation volume, form cakes with a porosity as high as 0.9. Since this is also associated with a decrease in specific surface, flocculation gives a marked increase in permeability. However, such coagulates are highly compressible and are therefore filtered at low pressures.

Filter aids are materials added in concentrations of up to 5% to slurries that filter only with difficulty. The filter aid forms a rigid cake of high porosity and permeability due to favorable shape characteristics, a low surface area, and a narrow particle size distribution, properties that can be varied for different operations. This structure mechanically supports the fine particles originally in the slurry. Diatomite, in the form of a purified, fractionated powder, is most commonly used. Other filter aids include a volcanic glass, called Perlite, and some cellulose derivatives.

Filter aids cannot easily be used when solids are wanted. Their excellent characteristics, however, lead to their use as a ''precoat'' mounted on a suitable support so that the filter aid itself forms the effective filtering medium. This prevents blinding the septum. Precoat methods take several forms and are discussed in Section 10.3.

## 10.2.5 Cake Compressibility

In the theory of cake filtration, the permeability coefficient was considered constant. The observation that a cake may be hard and firm at the cake septum junction and sloppy at its outer face suggests that the porosity may be varying throughout the cake depth. This variability could be due to decreased hydrostatic pressure from a maximum at the cake face to zero at the back of the supporting septum. The hydrostatic pressure must be balanced by a thrust, originating in the viscous drag of the fluid as it passes through the cake, transmitted through the cake skeleton, and varying from zero at the cake face to a maximum at the back of the septum equal to the pressure difference. The relation between this compressive stress and the pressure applied across the cake is represented in Figure 10.1.

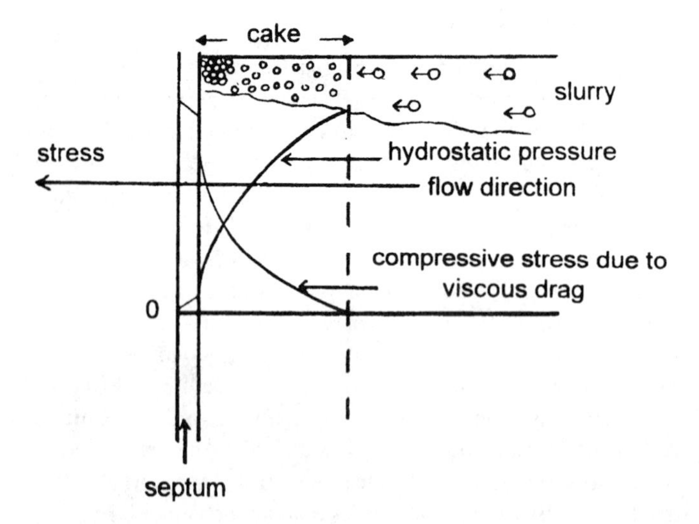


**FIGURE 10.1** Stress distribution in a filter cake.

We have so far considered that no deformation occurs under this stress; i.e., the cake is perfectly rigid. No cake, in fact, behaves in this way. However, some, such as those composed of filter aids or of coarse, isodiametric particles, approximate closely to a perfectly rigid cake. Others, such as cakes deposited from slurries of heavily hydrated colloidal particles, are easily deformed so that the permeability coefficient, until now assumed constant, is itself a function of pressure, so equation 10.1 no longer applies. This effect can be so marked that a pressure increase actually decreases the filtration rate. Most slurries' behavior is between these two extremes.

## 10.2.6 Cake Washing and Dewatering

Cake washing is of great importance in many filtration operations because the filtrate retained in the cake can be displaced by pure liquids. Filtration equipment varies in its washing efficiency, and this may influence the choice of plant. If the wash liquids follow the same course as the filtrate, the wash rate will be the same as the final rate of filtration, assuming that the viscosities of the two liquids are the same and that the cake structure is not altered by, for example, peptization following the removal of flocculating electrolytes. Washing takes place in two stages. The first involves removing most of the filtrate retained in the cake by simple displacement. In the second, longer stage, filtrate removal from the less accessible pores occurs by a diffusive mechanism. These stages are shown in Figure 10.2.

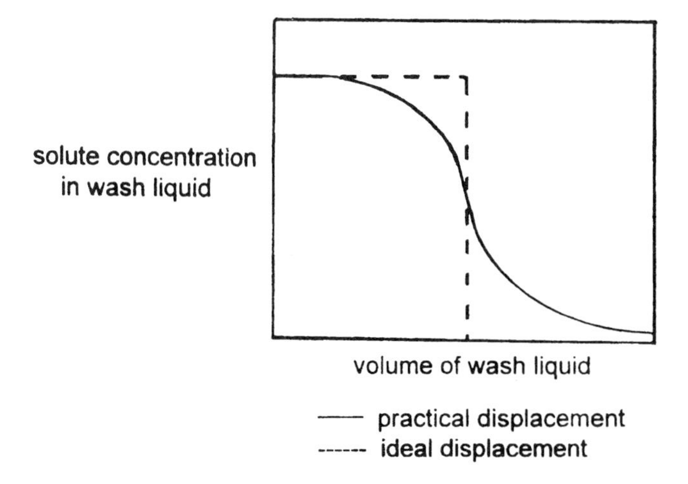


**FIGURE 10.2** Displacement of filtrate by displacement washing.

Efficient washing requires a fairly cohesive cake that opposes the formation of cracks and channels which offer a preferential course to the wash liquid. For this reason, cakes should have even thickness and permeability.

Subsequent operations, such as drying and handling, are facilitated by removing the liquid retained in the cake after washing, which occupies from 40% to 80% of the total cake volume. Removal is achieved by blowing or drawing air through the washed cake, leaving liquid retained only as a film around the particles and as annuli at the points of contact. Since surface area and the number of point contacts per unit volume increase as the particle size decreases, the effectiveness of this operation, like washing, decreases with cakes composed of fine particles.

## 10.3 FILTERS

The method by which filtrate is driven through the filter medium, and cake if present, is used to classify filters as follows:

1. Gravity filters
2. Vacuum filters
3. Pressure filters
4. The centrifuge

Each group may be further subdivided into filters employed in continuous or batch processes, although, due to technical difficulties, continuous pressure filters are uncommon and expensive. The general principles of each group are discussed and illustrated by several widely used filters.

### 10.3.1 Gravity Filters

Gravity filters employing thick, granular beds are widely used in municipal water filtration. However, the low operating pressures, usually less than $1.03 \times 10^4$ N/m$^2$, give low filtration rates unless very large areas are used. Their use in pharmacy is quite limited. Gravity filters using suspended media composed of thick felts are sometimes used for clarification on a small scale. On a somewhat larger scale, a wooden or stone tank, known as a *nutsche*, is used. The nutsche has a false bottom, which may act as the filter medium, although, more commonly, the bottom is dressed with a cloth. The slurry is added and the material filters under its own hydrostatic head. The filtrate is collected in the sump beneath the filter. Thorough washing is possible either by simple displacement and diffusion or by resuspending the solids in a wash liquid and refiltering. The nutsche is comparatively difficult to empty, and labor costs are high.

## 10.3.2 Vacuum Filters

Vacuum filters operate at higher pressure differentials than gravity filters. The pressure is limited naturally to about $8.27 \times 10^4$ N/m$^2$, which confines their use of vacuum filters to the deposition of fairly thin cakes of freely filtering materials. Despite this limitation, the principle has been successfully applied to continuous and completely automatic cake filtration, for which the rotary drum filter [Figure 10.3] is most extensively used. A typical construction may be regarded as two concentric, horizontal cylinders, the outer cylinder being the septum with a suitable perforated metal support. The annular space between the cylinders is divided by radial partitions producing a number of peripheral compartments running the length of the drum. Each compartment is connected by a line to a port in a rotary valve which permits the intermittent application of vacuum or compressed air as dictated by the different parts of

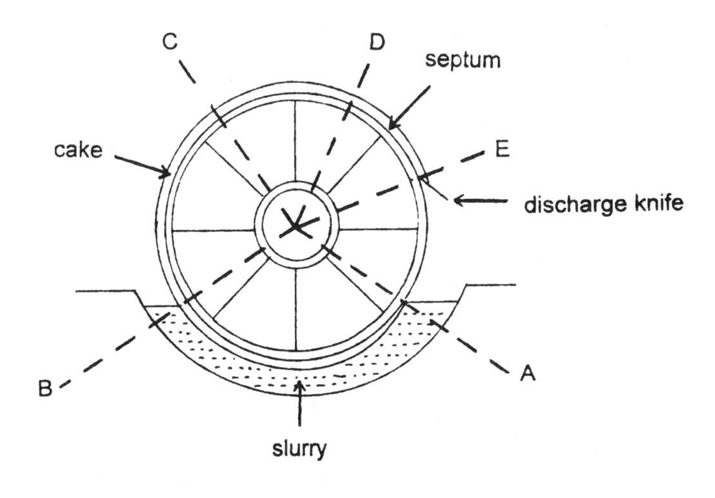


A-B Deposition of cake
C-D Washing
E Washing
B-C Cake drainage
D-E Partial drying

**FIGURE 10.3** Rotary vacuum filter.

the filtration cycle. The drum is partially immersed in a bath to which the slurry is fed. The complete cycle of filtration, washing, partial drying, and discharge is completed with each revolution of the drum and usually takes from 1 to 10 min. The relative lengths of each part of the cycle, indicated by the segments superimposed on the figure, depend on the cake-forming characteristics of the slurry and the importance of the associated operations of washing and drying. They may be varied by immersion depth and rotation speed so that each compartment remains submerged until an adequate cake is formed. Washing and dewatering can be carried out to the standard required during the remaining part of the cycle. The slurry must be effectively agitated during operation or sedimentation will cause the preferential deposition of the finer particles, giving a cake of low permeability. Agitation, of course, must not erode the deposited cake. Maintaining a suspension of very coarse particles, therefore, becomes difficult or impossible, and other methods of feeding must be adopted.

Filtration may be followed by a brief period of draining in which air is drawn through the cake, displacing retained filtrate. Washing is usually carried out with sprays, although devices which flood the cake have been used. Dewatering, again achieved by drawing air through the cake, is followed by discharge. A scraper knife, assisted by compressed air which causes the septum to belly against the cutting edge, is commonly used. Highly cohesive cakes, such as those encountered in the removal of mycelial growth from antibiotic cultures, may be removed by means of a string discharge. A series of closely spaced, parallel strings run on the cloth around the drum. At the discharge section the strings lift the cake away from the cloth and over a discharge roller after which the strings are led back to the drum.

Other variants of rotary drum filtration include top-feed filtration and precoat filtration. As mentioned, slurries containing coarse particles cannot be effectively suspended by the method described. Such materials, which give rapid cake formation and fast dewatering, may be filtered by applying the slurry to the top of the drum by using a feed box and suitable dams. Sedimentation in this case assists filtration.

Precoat filtration using a rotary drum is applied to slurries containing a small amount of fine or gelatinous material which plugs and blinds the filter cloth. Filtration is preceded by the deposition of a filter aid on the drum to a depth of up to 4 ins. Blinding of the surface layers occurs during filtration, but these layers are removed at the discharge section by a slowly advancing knife so that a clean filtering surface is continually presented to the slurry. The depth of cut depends on penetration of the precoat by the slurry solids and is usually about $10^{-5}$ m. This method has allowed the filtration of slurries which could not previously be filtered or which demanded the addition of large quantities of a filter aid.

For filtration on a smaller scale the nutsche is used. A vacuum is drawn on the sump of the tank, which gives a much faster filtration rate than in a gravity-operated process.

### 10.3.3 Pressure Filters

Due to the formation of low-permeability cakes, many slurries require higher-pressure differentials for effective filtration than can be applied by vacuum techniques. Pressure filters are used for such operations. They may also be used when the operation's scale does not justify installing continuous rotary filters. Usually, operational pressures of $6.89 \times 10^4$ to $6.89 \times 10^5$ N/m$^2$ are applied across stationary filter surfaces. This arrangement prohibits continuous operation because it is difficult to discharge the cake while the filter is under pressure. The higher labor costs of batch operation are, however, offset by lower capital costs.

The most commonly used pressure filter is the plate-and-frame filter press [Figure 10.4]. It consists of a series of alternating plates and frames mounted in line on bars which provide support and facilitate assembly and cake discharge. The filter cloth is mounted on the two faces of each plate, and

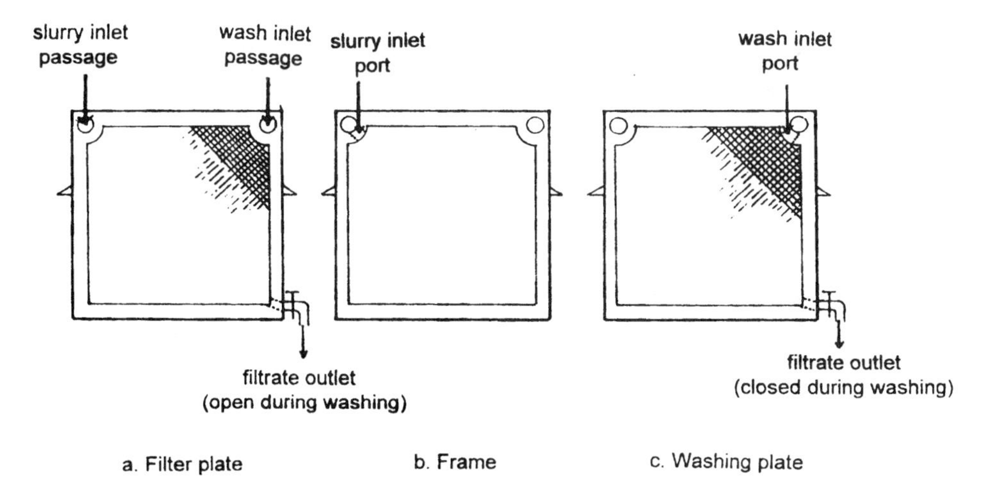


**FIGURE 10.4** The filter press: plates and frame.

the press is assembled by moving the plates and frames together with a hand screw or hydraulic ram. This provides a series of compartments, the peripheries of which are sealed by the machined edges of the plates and frames uniting on the filter cloth, which acts as a gasket. Dripping often occurs at this point, so the press is less suitable for noxious materials. The dimensions of each compartment are determined by the plate area and the intervening frame thickness. These dimensions and the number of compartments used depend primarily on the volume of slurry to be handled and its solids content. The plate faces are corrugated by grooves or ribs which effectively support the cloth, preventing distortion under pressure and allowing free discharge of the filtrate from behind the cloth. A section of the assembled filter press is given in Figure 10.5(a).

Coincident holes, shown in the top left-hand corner of both plates and frames, provide, on assembly, a channel for the slurry and, simultaneously, entry into each compartment through an entry port in each frame. All compart-

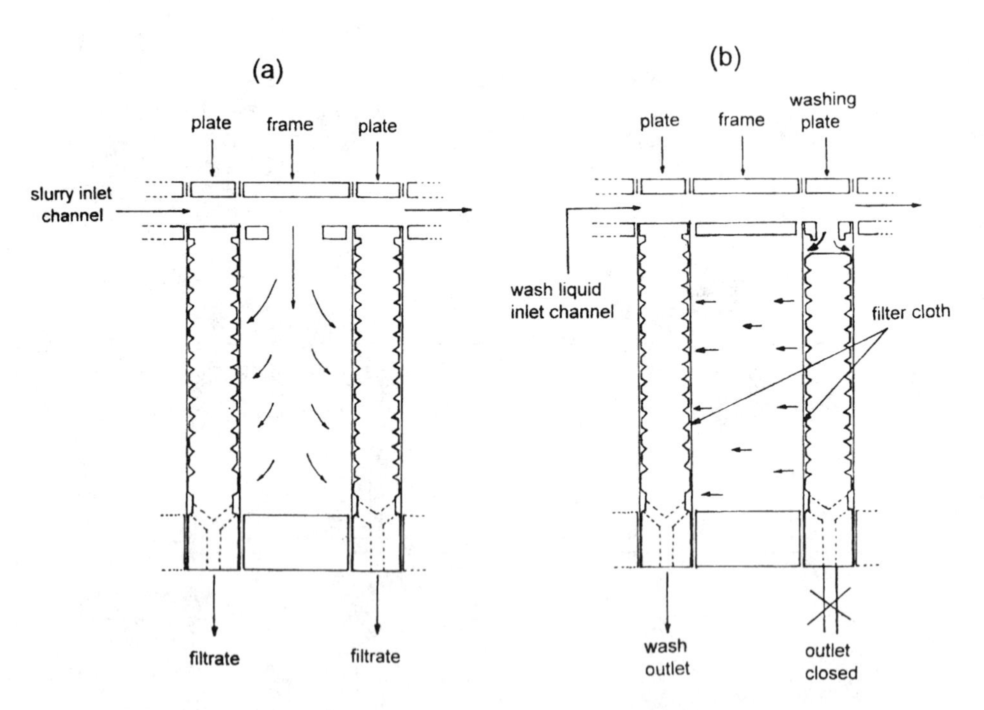


**FIGURE 10.5** Assembled filter press showing a frame and two plates. Movement of liquid during (a) filtration and (b) washing.

ments therefore behave in the same way with the formation of two cakes on the opposing plate faces. Discharge of filtrate after passage through cake, cloth, and corrugations takes place through an outlet in the plate shown diametrically opposite the frame entry port. Filtration may be continued until the cake entirely fills the compartments or the accumulation of cake gives unsatisfactory filtration rates.

Washing may be carried out by simply replacing the slurry with wash liquids and providing for its separate collection. This method, however, gives inefficient washing due to erosion and channeling of the cake. Where efficient washing is required, special washing plates alternate with the other plates described. These plates contain an additional inlet which leads the wash liquid in behind the filter cloth. During washing, the filtrate outlet on the washing plate is closed so that the wash liquid flows through the cloth and first cake in a direction opposite to that taken by the filtrate. The wash liquid then follows the course of the filtrate through the cake and cloth of the opposite plate. A diagram of liquid flow during washing is given in Figure 10.5(b).

The development of filter media in sheet form with high wet strength and the ability to retain extremely fine particles extends the application of the plate-and-frame filter to clarification. Such media occur in various grades and, when used in apparatus similar to that described, may be used to clarify or sterilize liquids containing a very low proportion of solids. In sterilization by sheet filtration, the operation is carried out in two stages. The solution is first clarified. The very clean filtrate is then passed through the sterilizing sheet under a relatively low pressure. Before the operation, the assembled filter is sterilized by steam. The washing apparatus, assembled with suitable sheets, may also be used for air filtration.

Other filters widely used for clarification are the Metafilter and the Streamline filter. The former consists of numerous closely spaced rings, usually made of stainless steel, mounted on a rod. The rod is fluted to provide channels for filtrate discharge. The passage of filtrate between the rings is provided by scallops stamped on one side of each ring which maintain a ring spacing of between $1 \times 10^{-5}$ and $8 \times 10^{-5}$ m. This construction provides a robust support for the actual filtering medium. It is mounted in a suitable pressure vessel, and large filters consist of several units. For clarification the filter is first coated by circulating filter aid of the correct grade. The finest materials are suitable for bacteria removal. The coat acts as a depth filter. Filter aids may also be added to the liquid to be clarified.

The Streamline filter employs paper disks compressed to form a filter pack. The filtrate passes through the minute interstices between the disks, leaving any solids at the edge. This is the principle of edge filtration. Other filters, composed of metal plates or wires, operate on the same principle and are used for coarse clarification.

Many small-scale filters consist simply of a fixed, rigid medium, robust enough to withstand limited pressures, mounted in a suitable housing. Such filters, which are also vacuum-operated, are used to clarify by depth filtration. Media are composed of sintered metals, ceramics, plastics, or glass. Filters prepared from closely graded and sintered ceramic powders are suitable for sterilizing solutions by filtration on a manufacturing scale.

## 10.4 FILTER MEDIA

The choice of filter medium for a particular operation demands considerable experience. In clarification, high filtration rates and the retention of fine particles are opposing requirements. Permeability and retentive capacity can be determined and used to guide small-scale experiments with the materials to be filtered, facilities for which are often made available by filter manufacturers. Other relevant factors are filtrate contamination by the medium and associated housing, adsorption of materials from solutions, and, where necessary, the medium's ability to withstand repeated sterilization.

In cake filtration the medium must oppose excessive penetration and promote the formation of a junction with the cake of high permeability. The medium should also give free discharge of cake after washing and dewatering.

### 10.4.1 Rigid Media

Rigid media may be loose or fixed. The former is exemplified by the deposition of a filter aid on a suitable support. Filtration characteristics are governed mainly by particle size, size distribution, and shape as described earlier. These factors may be varied for different filtering requirements.

Fixed media vary from perforated metals used for coarse straining to removal of very fine particles with a sintered aggregate of metal, ceramic, plastic, or glass powder. The size, size distribution, and shape of the powder particles together with the sintering conditions control the size and distribution of the pores in the final product. The permeability may be expressed in terms of the constant in equation 10.1. Alternatively, the medium may be characterized by air permeability. The maximum pore size, which is important when selecting filters for sterilization, may be determined by measuring the pressure difference required to blow a bubble of air through the medium while it supports a column of liquid with a known surface tension.

### 10.4.2 Flexible Media

Flexible media may be woven or unwoven. Filter media woven from cotton, wool, synthetic and regenerated fibers, glass, and metal fibers are used as septa in cake filtration. Cotton is most widely used, and nylon is predominant among synthetic fibers. Terylene is a useful medium for acid filtration. Penetration and cake discharge are influenced by the way in which fibers are twisted and plied and by the adoption of various weaves such as duck and twill. The choice of a cloth often depends on the chemical nature of the slurry.

Nonwoven media occur in the form of felts and compressed cellulose pulps and are used for clarification by depth filtration. A disadvantage, unless the medium is carefully prepared, is the loss of fibrous material from the filter's downstream side. The application of sheet media has already been discussed. High wet strength is conferred on paper sheets by resin impregnation. An alternative manufacture employs asbestos fibers supported in a cellulose framework.

## 10.5 AIR FILTRATION

Removing particulate matter from air along with controlling humidity, temperature, and distribution is the purpose of air conditioning. Solid and liquid particles are most commonly arrested by filtration, although other methods, such as electrostatic precipitation, cyclones, and scrubbers, are used in some circumstances. The objective may be simply to provide comfortable and healthy conditions for work, or it may be dictated by the operations proceeding in the area. Some industrial processes demand large volumes of clean air.

This section is concerned mainly with air filtration, the objective of which is the reduction or complete removal of bacteria. This is applied, with varying stringency, to several operations associated with pharmacy. Where sterilization is the objective and the presence of inanimate particles is of secondary importance, other methods, such as ultraviolet radiation and heating, must be added.

Bacteria rarely exist singly in the atmosphere but are usually associated with much larger particles. For example, it has been shown that 78% of particles carrying *C. welchii* were greater than $4.2 \times 10^{-6}$ m. The average diameter exceeded $10 \times 10^{-6}$ m. On this basis it has been suggested that air filters which are 99.9% efficient at $5 \times 10^{-6}$ m are adequate for filtering air supplied to operating theaters and dressing wards. On the other hand, filters used to clean air supplied to large-scale aerobic fermentation cultures must offer a very low probability that any organism will penetrate during the process. This became important in the deep culture production of penicillin when the ingress of a single penicillinase-producing organism could be disastrous. Similarly, stringent conditions are laid down for the air supply to areas where sterile products are prepared and handled.

### 10.5.1 Mechanism of Air Filtration

A theoretical foundation for air filtration by passage through fibrous media was laid in the early 1930s by studies of the flow of suspended particles around various obstacles. In studies of the filtration of smokes (Hinds, 1982) it has been shown that the following five factors operate simultaneously in arresting a particle during its passage through a filter, although their relative importance varies with the type of filter and the conditions under which it is operated.

1. Diffusion effects due to Brownian movement
2. Electrostatic attraction between particles and fibers
3. Direct interception of a particle by a fiber
4. Interception as a result of inertial effects acting on a particle and causing it to collide with a fiber
5. Settling and gravitational effects

Air filters operate under conditions of streamline flow, as indicated by the streamlines drawn around a cylindrical fiber in cross section in Figure 10.6. It was assumed that particle capture takes place if any contact is made during the particle movement around the fiber. Once capture occurs, the particle is not reentrained in the airstream but is deposited deeper in the bed. Never-

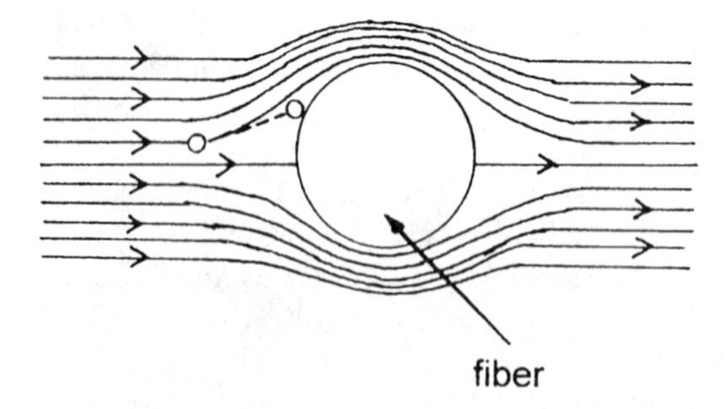


**FIGURE 10.6** Inertial capture of a particle by a fiber.

theless, some fiber filters are treated with viscous oils, presumably to make capture more positive and to reduce reentrainment.

If a particle remains in a streamline while passing around the fiber, capture occurs only if the particle radius exceeds the distance between streamline and fiber, a dimension dependent on the particle and fiber diameters. This mechanism, termed *capture by direct interception*, is independent of the air velocity except insofar as the streamlines are modified by changes in air velocity.

Deviation of particles from streamlines can occur in various ways (Hinds, 1982). The chance of capture increases if Brownian movement causes appreciable migration across streamlines, an effect important only for small particles (less than $5 \times 10^{-7}$ m) and low air speeds, when the time spent in the vicinity of a fiber is relatively large. These conditions also apply to capture which is the result of electrostatic attraction.

The inertial mechanism depends on particle mass, fiber diameter, and approach velocity. The particle deviates from the streamline and follows the broken line in Figure 10.6. Capture occurs if the deviation, which increases as the mass and velocity of the particle increase, brings the particle into contact with the fiber.

The simultaneous operation of mechanisms, at least one of which demands low air speeds and fine particles for effectiveness and another which requires large particles traveling at high speeds, suggests that maximum penetration could occur at an intermediate air speed. Conversely, there is, for any given conditions, an optimal particle size for which the combined filtration effects are a minimum and penetration is a maximum. A diagram of the mechanism interaction is reproduced in Figure 10.7. Similar effects were demon-

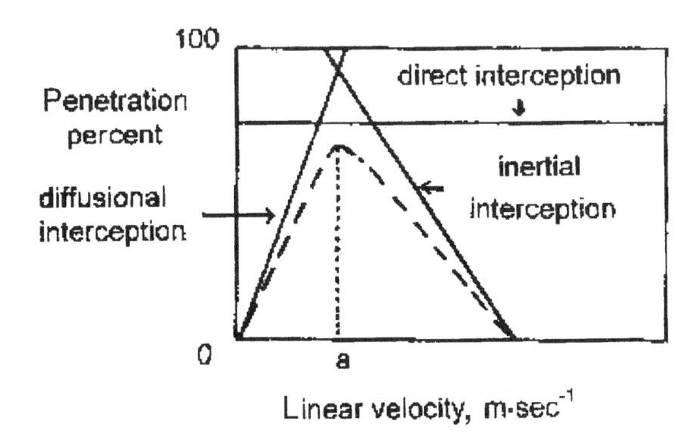


**FIGURE 10.7** Interaction of the mechanisms of particle arrest.

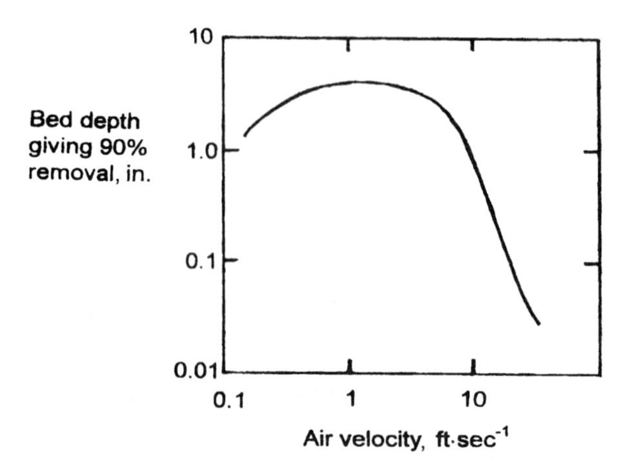


**FIGURE 10.8** Effect of airstream velocity on bacterial spores removal by a filter.

strated for bacterial aerosols by Humphrey and Gaden, who estimated the efficiency with which a glass fiber mat collected *B. subtilis* spores atomized as particles just over a micron in radius. The results are presented in Figure 10.8. A theoretical approach to the removal of industrial dusts has been developed by Stairmand and Fuchs.

### 10.5.2 The Design, Operation, and Testing of Air Filters

Granular beds, fibrous media, and absolute filters prepared from cellulose and asbestos are used for high-efficiency air filtration. With fibrous and granular filters, the fractional reduction in particle content is assumed to be the same through successive incremental thicknesses of the filter. We may therefore rewrite equation 10.2 as

$$\frac{dC}{dx} = -kC \tag{10.2}$$

where $C$ represents the number of particles entering a section of thickness $dx$. The constant $k$ is a measure of the filter's ability to retain a particle and is a complex function of fiber diameter, interfiber distance, and the operational air velocity. Integration between inlet and outlet conditions gives

$$\log \frac{C_{\text{out}}}{C_{\text{in}}} = -kx \tag{10.3}$$

If a certain filter thickness is capable of retaining 90% of the entering particles, then, if $10^6$ particles enter, $10^5$ will penetrate. If six thicknesses are used, then the preceding relation predicts that only one particle penetrates. The log-penetration effect has been confirmed for fibrous filters and for granular beds. It must be stressed, however, that fibrous and granular filters present passages very much greater than the fine particles they remove. Absolute sterility or absolute filtration at a certain particle size cannot be achieved. However, design variables, such as fiber diameter, fiber packing density, filter thickness, and air speed. For example, these variables may be varied to give air which, for a given input contamination, is, with a high statistical probability, sterile.

In an early study, Terjesen and Cherryl used a bacterial aerosol and a Bourdillon slit sampler to test the suitability of filters for air sterilization. They showed that 0.075-m slabs of slag wool composed of fibers, most of which were less than $6 \times 10^{-6}$ m and compressed to a suitable density, gave sterile air when operated for 15 days at a face velocity of 0.152 m $s^{-1}$. A similar efficiency was found for filters composed of glass fibers of similar diameters. Resin-bonded filter mats composed of glass fibers $12 \times 10^{-6}$–$13 \times 10^{-6}$ m in diameter have also been described. An assembly of these mats to give a filter 0.304 m deep effectively removes bacteria.

Bacteria may be effectively removed by passing air through deep granular beds of activated carbon, alumina, and other materials. Table 10.1 gives data on the efficiency of alumina in a bed 0.381 m deep for removing *Serratia marcescens* from air. The effect of two design variables, granule size and air speed, is illustrated.

**Table 10.1** Removal of *Seratia marcescens* with a 0.3-m Bed of Alumina Granules

| Air velocity (m/min) | Efficiency (percent removal) | |
|---|---|---|
| | 8–16 mesh | 16–32 mesh |
| 24.4 | — | 92 |
| 73.2 | 88 | 99.4 |
| 146.3 | 98.7 | 99.9 |
| 219.5 | 99.86 | — |

The extremely hazardous nature of radioactive dusts has promoted the design of high-efficiency air filters for use where such materials are handled. These filters may be used for any application requiring extremely pure air. A medium in paper form was constructed from cellulose and asbestos. This could be pleated round corrugated spacers to give a large filtering area in a relatively small space. A paper composed of very fine glass fibers was later developed which resisted temperatures up to 773 K and could, therefore, be sterilized.

The general object of all filter design is the virtual certainty of removing the particles under consideration with a medium offering minimal resistance to airflow. Unlike liquid clarifiers, air filters become more efficient with time because accumulation of particles restricts passage through the medium. This deposition causes an increase in the pressure differential required to maintain a given flow rate. When the filter has become laden with a certain amount of dust, it must be cleaned or replaced. The life of high-efficiency air filters may be lengthened by first passing the air through a coarse, or ''roughing,'' filter which removes the largest particles.

The use of bacterial aerosols as tracer organisms to test filter efficiency has already been described. Other tests with inanimate dusts are more generally used to evaluate filter performance. For general ventilation purposes two tests are specified. The first determines gravimetrically the capacity of the filter to hold dust and still function satisfactorily. A standard dust of $5 \times 10^{-6}$ or $26 \times 10^{-5}$ m is passed into the filter until a specified increase in airflow resistance occurs. The second test, which is also applicable to high-efficiency filters, determines the fraction of a methylene blue aerosol which passes through the filter under given conditions. The aerosol is generated by atomizing a 1% aqueous solution of methylene blue. The droplets dry to give a cloud of particles, 90% of which are below $2 \times 10^{-7}$ m. The test is therefore extremely stringent. The cloud is passed through the filter at a constant rate ($10^{-3}$ $m^3$ $min^{-1}$) and then through a strip of porous paper that collects any methylene blue particles which have penetrated. The stain due to the dye, after intensification in steam, is compared to a series of similar stains which correspond to known volumes of unfiltered air. Thus, if $60 \times 10^{-3}$ $m^3$ of filtered air give a stain which matches that produced by $1.2 \times 10^{-5}$ $m^3$ of unfiltered air, the penetration is 0.02%. An alternative method of evaluating penetration employs a cloud produced by the atomization of a solution of sodium chloride. After passage through the filter, part of the air is passed through a hydrogen flame. The intensity of the sodium flame produced is estimated with a photoelectric cell.

## 10.6 THE CENTRIFUGE

An object moving in a circular path is subjected to an outward centrifugal force which balances the centripetal force moving the object toward the center of rotation. This principle is used in the mechanical separations called centrifugal filtration and centrifugal sedimentation. In the former, a material is placed in a rotating perforated basket lined with a filter cloth. This material is used to separate a solid, which is retained at the cloth, from a liquid. It is essentially a filtration process in which the driving force is of centrifugal origin. It in no way depends on a difference in the density of the two phases.

In centrifugal sedimentation the separation is due to the difference in the density of two or more phases. In this more important process, solid-liquid mixtures and liquid-liquid mixtures can be completely separated. If, however, the separation is incomplete, there will be a gradient in the size of the dispersed phase within the centrifuge due to the faster radial velocity of the larger particles. Operated in this way the centrifuge becomes a classifier.

### 10.6.1 Centrifugal Filtration

The filtration principles discussed previously can be directly applied to centrifugal filtration, although theoretical predictions of filtration rate and spinning time are uncertain. The process is widely used for separating crystals and granular products from other liquors, but it is less effective if the slurry contains a high proportion of particles less than $1 \times 10^{-4}$ m. The advantages of the process are effective washing and drying. Residual moisture after centrifugation is far less than in cakes produced by pressure or vacuum filtration. By this method the moisture content of a cake of coarse crystals can be reduced to as low as 3%. This facilitates the drying operation which normally follows. Enclosure of the centrifuge is easy so that toxic and volatile materials can be processed.

A typical batch filter [Figure 10.9(a)] consists of a perforated metal basket mounted on a vertical axis. The cloth used to retain solids is often supported on a metal screen Baskets mounted as shown are emptied by shoveling the cake. If, however, top suspension is used, the cake can be more easily withdrawn through traps in the base of the basket. In batch operation considerable time is lost during machine acceleration and deceleration. Machines operating with continuous discharge of solids are used for separating coarse solids during large-scale operations. Such machines are commonly constructed with a horizontal axis of rotation.

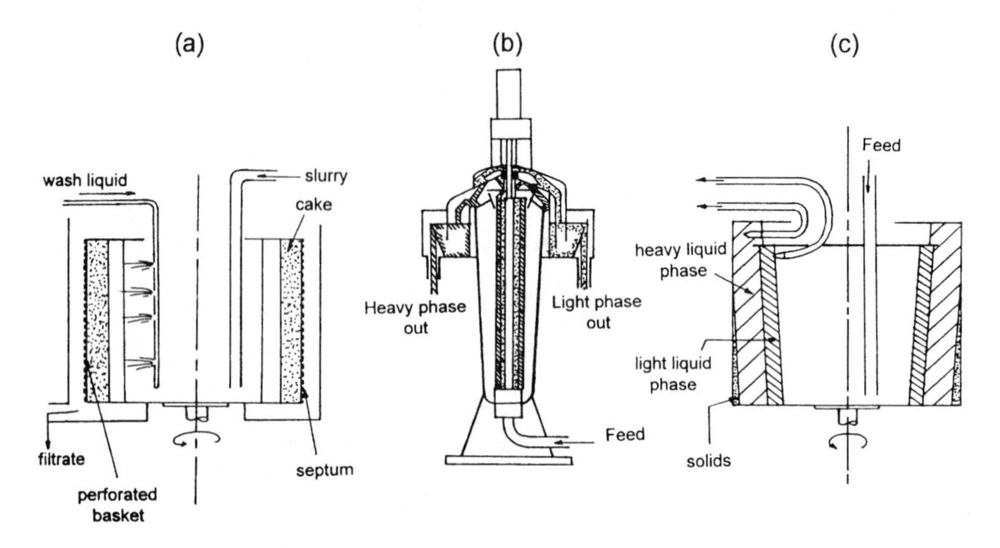


**FIGURE 10.9** (a) Batch centrifugal filter, (b) supercentrifuge, and (c) solid bowl batch centrifuge.

## 10.6.2 Centrifugal Sedimentation

Particle motion in a liquid is described by Stokes' equation. If its diameter is $d$, the rate, $u$, at which it settles by gravity in a liquid of viscosity $\eta$ and density $\rho$ is given by equation 1.24:

$$u = \frac{1}{18} d^2 \frac{\rho_p - \rho}{\eta} g \tag{1.24}$$

where $g$ in acceleration due to gravity and $\rho_p$ is the particle density. In the centrifuge the gravitational force causing separation is replaced by a centrifugal force. If the particle has a mass $m$ and moves at an angular velocity $\omega$ in a circle of radius $r$, the centrifugal force is $\omega^2 r(m - m_1)$, where $m_1$ is the mass of the displaced liquid. Therefore, $\omega^2 r/g$ is the ratio of the centrifugal and gravitational forces in the given example. Its value can exceed 10,000. The separation is, therefore, quicker, more complete, and more effective in systems containing very fine particles that will not sediment by gravity because of Brownian movement.

Expressing the particle mass in terms of its volume and effective density, we can write the centrifugal force as

$$\frac{\pi}{6} d^2(\rho_g - \rho)\omega^2 r \tag{10.4}$$

In streamline conditions the opposing viscous force, given by equation 1.22, is $3\pi d\eta u$, $u$ being the terminal velocity of the particle. Equating these expressions gives

$$u = \frac{1}{18} d^2\left(\frac{\rho_g - \rho}{\eta}\right)\omega^2 r \tag{10.5}$$

The sedimentation rate is proportional to the radius of the basket and the square of the speed at which it rotates. Centrifugal sedimentors can be divided into various types.

For operation at very high speeds, the centrifuge bowl is tubular with a length-diameter ratio from 4 to 8. An example is the Sharples supercentrifuge [Figure 10.9(b)] which operates at up to 15,000 rpm or, in turbine-driven laboratory models, up to 50,000 rpm. The machine, which gives continuous discharge of two separated liquids, is widely used in emulsion separation. It is also an effective clarifier when the concentration of solids is very low. These are periodically discharged by scraping the walls of the centrifuge tube. Uses include cleaning fats and waxes, blood fractionation, and virus recovery.

Disk-type centrifuges introduce baffles into the bowl in order to decrease the distance which particles travel before settling at the wall. They split the liquid into layers in which separation occurs. The length-to-diameter ratio is usually much smaller than in tubular bowl centrifuges and operational speeds are lower. In batch processes the machine is discharged manually at intervals. Larger machines continuously or intermittently discharge the solids as a thick slurry through nozzles or valves at the basket periphery.

A solid bowl batch basket is shown in Figure 10.9(c). In this type of machine liquids are discharged by weirs or skimmers. Two skimmers are shown, each taking off a liquid phase. Solids are discharged manually at the end of the process. In continuous models a conveying scroll, operating at a slightly different speed from the basket, plows the solids to one end and discharges the material as a damp powder.

# 11

# Size Reduction and Classification

## 11.1 THE IMPORTANCE OF FINE PARTICLES IN PHARMACY

Although fine particles can be produced directly by controlled precipitation, by crystallization, or by drying a fine spray of solution, in many cases the material is powdered in some kind of mill. From our point of view, the most important result of this operation is the increase in surface area of a given weight of the powder and its influence on diffusional processes. A cube of side 0.01 m has a surface area of $6 \times 10^{-4}$ m$^2$. If, by some ideal size reduction process, this cube was divided into cubes of side 0.001 m, we would have a thousand particles each with a surface area of $6 \times 10^{-6}$ m$^2$, and a total surface area of $6 \times 10^{-3}$ m$^2$. A 10-fold increase in surface area has been given by a 10-fold decrease in particle size. Generalizing, we may say that the surface area is inversely proportional to the particle size, assuming that the particle shape remains the same.

The rate of most chemical and physical reactions involving solids and liquids is greatly influenced by the area of interfacial contact. In chemical reactions a reagent must diffuse toward the surface of the solid, the reaction products must diffuse away, a procedure which depends, among other things, on the area between solid and liquid. The effect of particle size on dissolution rate exemplifies another aspect of diffusion which is important to the pharmacist. Most commonly, drugs are taken orally in the form of solid particles, and absorption, which is usually rapid, must be preceded by dissolution. A full discussion of the role of particle size in oral, parenteral, and topical therapy may be found in Newman and Axon (1961) and Wagner (1961).

The rate at which fine chemicals or drugs are extracted from a vegetable source is increased by an increase in surface area. Reducing particle size increases the area available for materials transfer and decreases the distance over which solvent and solute must diffuse; it also has a marked effect on drying porous materials.

Other effects, not based on diffusion and its dependence on surface area, are found in mixing and various formulation requirements. If we withdraw a sample from a mixture of powders, it is unlikely to contain exactly the correct proportion of ingredients. However, the larger the number of particles in the sample, the closer the sample will represent the overall proportions of the mixture. We can therefore increase the sample accuracy which might eventually form a tablet or a capsule, by increasing the number of particles it contains—that is, reduce the particle size of the mix components. Since difference of particle size promotes segregation, the components should be produced with a similar particle size distribution.

Formulation requirements often dictate the use of fine particles. Impalpability and spreading are required of dusting and cosmetic powders. Particles of $3.5 \times 10^{-5}$–$4.0 \times 10^{-5}$ m can be detected as single particles when applied to the skin and may give the impression of grittiness. Such powders should, in general, be finer than $3.0 \times 10^{-5}$ m. When powders are tinted, the particle size of powder and pigment affect the final color. In tableting, careful size reduction of imperfect tablets provides a material suitable for compression. The flow properties of suspensions of high disperse phase concentration is affected by particle size and size distribution. At a given disperse phase concentration, decreasing particle size leads to increasing viscosity, whereas broadening the particle size distribution leads to decreasing viscosity. Sedimentation is a function of particle size.

Numerous examples have been quoted to stress the importance of fine particles in pharmacy. Milling or grinding offers a method by which these particles may be produced, size classification gives a means, where applicable, of selecting a desired fraction or of removing oversize or undersize particles, and size analysis provides the analytical tool by which these operations may be assessed and controlled.

## 11.2 FUNDAMENTAL ASPECTS OF CRUSHING AND GRINDING

A basic study of crushing and grinding considers the physical properties of the material, the crushing mechanism itself, and its relation to the mechanism of failure. When a stress, which may be compressive, tensile, or shear, is applied to a solid, the latter deforms. Initially, the deformation or strain is the distortion of the crystal lattice by relative displacement of its components without change of structure. Complete recovery follows stress removal, and behavior is elastic. Figure 11.1 considers the deformation of a solid under a tensile stress, and elastic behavior is shown over section AB. Below the elastic limit (B) stress is proportional to strain and is related to it by various moduli. Beyond the yield point (C) permanent or plastic deformation occurs, and, as shown by release of stress at point D, all strain is not recoverable. Sliding along natural cleavage planes is occurring in this region. Plastic deformation is terminated by failure or fracture, which is normally a quite gradual and reproducible process preceded by material thinning. The stress at point E is a measure of the material's strength. The area under the curve at any point represents the strain energy per unit volume absorbed by the specimen up to that strain. The limiting strain energy per unit volume is the energy absorbed up to the point of failure.

An extensive period of plastic deformation is shown in Figure 11.1, and the material would be classified as ductile. For the brittle materials normally encountered in grinding, little plastic deformation takes place and the points C and E almost coincide. Fracture is here explained in terms of cracks and

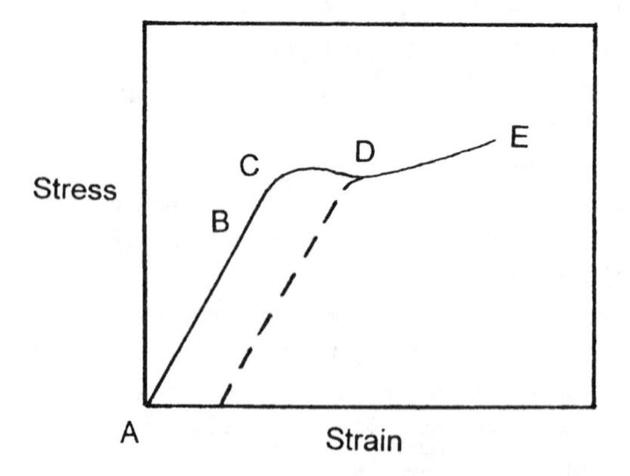


**FIGURE 11.1** Tensile deformation of a ductile material.

flaws naturally present in the material. It occurs suddenly and with shattering. The energy employed in stressing the particle to the point of failure reappears mainly as heat on release of strain in a manner analogous to the sudden release of a stressed spring.

The theoretical strength of crystalline materials can be calculated from interatomic attractive and repulsive forces. The strength of real materials, however, is found to be many times smaller than the theoretical value. The discrepancy is explained in terms of flaws of various kinds, such as minute fissures or irregularities of lattice structure known as *dislocations*. They have the capacity to concentrate the stress in the vicinity of the flaw. Failure may then occur at a much lower overall stress than is predicted from the theoretical considerations. Failure occurs with the development of a crack tip which propagates rapidly through the material while penetrating other flaws which may, in turn, produce secondary cracks. The strength of the material therefore depends on the random distribution of flaws and is a statistical quantity varying within fairly wide limits. This concept explains why a material becomes progressively more difficult to grind. Since the probability of containing an effective flaw decreases as particle size decreases, the strength increases until, with the achievement of faultless domains, the material strength equals the theoretical strength. This position is not realized in practice due to complicating factors such as aggregation.

The strength of most materials is greater in compression than in tension. It is therefore unfortunate that technical difficulties prevent the direct use of tensile stresses. The compressive stresses commonly used in comminution equipment do not cause failure directly but generate, by distortion, sufficient tensile or shear stress to form a crack tip in a region away from the point of primary stress application. This mechanism is inefficient but unavoidable. Impact and attrition are the other basic modes of stress application. The distinction between impact and compression is referred to later. Attrition, which is commonly employed, is difficult to classify but is probably primarily a shear mechanism.

In any machine one mode of stress application usually predominates. It must be correctly chosen with respect to the mechanical properties of the material. Compression, for example, is useless for comminution of fibrous or waxy solids. Attrition is generally necessary for all fine grinding.

The deformation and subsequent failure of a brittle material are not only a function of stress but also of the rate at which the stress is applied. Different results may be obtained from slow compressive breaking and impact breaking at the same energy. Particle shape, size, and size distribution may be affected. In impact breaking the rate of stress application is so high that the limiting strain energy may be exceeded several times by the suddenness of the operation. The reason is that fracture is time dependent, with a lag occurring between the application of maximum stress and failure.

Stress application is further complicated by ''free-crushing'' and ''packed-crushing'' mechanisms. In free crushing, the stress is applied to an unconstrained particle and released when failure occurs. In packed crushing, the application of stress continues on the crushed bed of particles. Although further size reduction occurs, the process is less efficient due to vitiation of energy by the effects of interparticulate friction and stress transmission via particles which do not themselves fracture. This is easily demonstrated when a crystalline material is ground in a pestle and mortar. The fine powder initially produced protects coarser particles. If the material is sieved and oversize particles returned, the operation may be completed with far less effort.

Free crushing is most nearly approached in the roller mill, which explains the high efficiency of the machine, and, to a lesser extent, in other continuous processes in which individual particles are presented to the grinding media. Packed crushing occurs in ball mills.

## 11.3 GRINDING EFFICIENCY

Extensive investigation of the relation between the energy supplied to a mill and the size reduction achieved has been carried out. The efficiency of the process reflected by such a relation is of small importance in pharmacy because the applications are limited. For completeness, however, they will be considered.

Most of the energy supplied to the mill is ultimately dissipated as heat due to mechanical inefficiency. Most of the remainder or net grinding energy also appears as heat produced on the release of strain energy, a small part being added to the internal energy of the system as, for example, surface energy.

Various hypotheses relate the net grinding energy applied to a process and the size reduction achieved. The first, proposed by Karl von Rittinger in 1867, states that the energy necessary for size reduction is directly proportional to the increase in surface area:

$$E = k(S_p - S_f) \quad (11.1)$$

where $E$ is the energy consumed, and $S_p$ and $S_f$ are the surface area of product and feed materials, respectively. The constant $k$ depends on the grinding unit employed and represents the energy consumed in enlarging the surface area by one unit. The relation between surface area and particle size has already been derived, and we may therefore write

$$E = k'\left(\frac{1}{d_p} - \frac{1}{d_f}\right) \tag{11.2}$$

where $d_f$ and $d_p$ are the particle sizes of feed and product particles, respectively.

The hypothesis indicates that energy consumption per unit area of new surface produced increases faster than the linear ratio of feed and product dimensions, a phenomenon already noted and explained. The proportionality of net energy input and new surface produced has been confirmed in some grinding operations.

Although Rittinger's law is concerned with surfaces and not with the energy associated with those surfaces, it is rational to relate crushing energy consumed and the surface energy gained by increase of surface area, thereby arriving at a measure of efficiency. In experiments in which single particles are crushed, between 1% and 30% of the applied energy appears as surface energy. In practical systems, when application of stress is less ideal, the net grinding energy is 100 to 1000 times greater than that associated with the new surface; i.e., the efficiency of the process, on this basis, is between 0.1% and 1%.

The relation of energy to surface area provides little information on the grinding process and does not influence mill design. It provides, however, the basis of some grindability tests in which a known amount of energy is supplied to a mill and the increase in surface is measured. This application is restricted to fine grinding.

Conversion of grinding energy to surface energy is neglected in Kick's law, enunciated in 1885. The law is based on the deformation and brittle failure of elastic bodies and states that the energy required to produce analogous changes of configuration of geometrically similar bodies is proportional to the weight or volume of those bodies. The energy requirements are independent of the initial particle size; they depend only on the size reduction ratio. Kick's law predicts lower energies than Rittinger's relation. The theory, however, demands that the resistance to crushing not change with particle size. The role of flaws present in real materials is not considered, with the result that the energy required for fine grinding, when the apparent strength may have greatly risen, is underestimated.

A third theory of comminution, put forth by Bond, gives results intermediate between the predictions of the laws of Kick and Rittinger. The theory rests upon three principles, the first of which states that any divided material must have a positive energy register. This can only be zero when the particle size becomes infinite. The input energy, $E$, for any size reduction process then equals the product energy register minus the feed energy register. The energy associated with a powder increases as the particle size decreases, and we may assume that the energy register is inversely proportional to the particle size to an exponent, $n$. Hence,

$$E = E_{\mathrm{p}} - E_{\mathrm{f}} = \frac{K}{d_{\mathrm{p}}^{\mathrm{n}}} - \frac{K}{d_{\mathrm{f}}^{\mathrm{n}}} \tag{11.3}$$

The second principle of Bond's theory assigns to $n$ a value of $i$, stating that ''the total work useful in breaking which has been applied to a stated weight of an homogeneous material is inversely proportional to the square root of the diameter of the product particles.''

The third principle states that material breakage is determined by the flaw structure. This aspect of size reduction has already been discussed.

An empirical, but realistic, approach to mill efficiency is gained through experiments in which the energy consumed and size reduction achieved are compared with values obtained in a laboratory test operating under free-crushing conditions. All energy supplied in the latter is available for crushing, and the test is assumed to be 100% efficient. Both slow-crushing and impact tests are used. Many single particles may be simultaneously crushed, and the work done may be measured. The latter is then related to the size reduction achieved. Similar measurements can be made during practical milling, expressing the efficiency of the process as a percentage of the free-crushing value. On this basis, approximate efficiency of the roll crusher is 80%, the swing hammer mill is 40%, the ball mill is 10%, and the fluid energy mill is only 1%.

## 11.4 OPERATION OF MILLS

In some operations, such as those in which ores are processed, size reduction may constitute a major proportion of total process costs. The efficiency with which energy is utilized is, therefore, of great importance. Drugs, on the other hand, fall into a class of materials which is expensive and processed in relatively small quantities. The contribution of grinding to total costs is, therefore, smaller, and the choice of machine can usually be made on technological rather than economic grounds. Generally, drugs are easy to grind. The operation is classified as fine, grinding if the bulk of the product passes a 200 mesh screen

($7.6 \times 10^{-5}$ m), or as superfine grinding, if a powder of a few microns or less is required. Most pharmaceutical grinding falls into these classes, although coarser grinding is applied to vegetable drugs before extraction.

Heywood stated that any type of crushing or grinding machine exhibits optimal comminution conditions for which the ratio of the energy to new surface is minimal (Heywood, 1957). If finer grinding is attempted in such a machine, the ratio is increased. Mills may thus become grossly inefficient if called upon to grind at a size for which they were not designed. A limited size reduction ratio is imposed on a single operation, larger ratios being obtained by the adoption of several stages, each employing a suitable mill. The fluid energy mill, which presents a size reduction ratio of up to 400, is exceptional.

A low retention time is inherent in free-crushing machines. Little overgrinding takes place, and the production of excessive undersize material or "fines" is avoided. Protracted milling times are found with many slow-speed mills, with the result that considerable overgrinding takes place. Accumulation of product particles within the mill reduces the effectiveness of breaking stresses, and the efficiency of milling progressively decreases. This is typical of "open-circuit" grinding, in which the material is passed only once through the mill and remains until virtually all has reached the required product size. An overall increase in efficiency is secured in "closed-circuit" grinding. Product particles are removed from the mill by means of a current of air or liquid by screens. The removed product may then be classified and any oversize material returned to the mill. Adoption of closed-circuit grinding techniques is only possible on a relatively large scale. On a smaller scale the effect can be simulated by periodic classification of the entire mill contents and the removal of material which has reached the required size.

### 11.4.1 Dry and Wet Grinding

Between the approximate limits of 5% and 50% moisture, materials cake and do not flow. Both factors oppose effective grinding. Dry grinding is carried out at low moisture contents, the upper limit depending on the nature of the material. Although 5% or more moisture may be permissible for vegetable drugs, it would prove excessive during the milling of a coarse, impervious solid.

Wet grinding is a common procedure when a fluid suspension is required, and drying, which would prove a significant drawback, is unnecessary. An excellent dispersion can be produced simultaneously, and, in some operations, this provides the primary objective, size reduction being of secondary importance. Wet grinding may also be adopted when the size reduction achieved during dry grinding is prematurely limited by aggregation.

Certain general advantages are secured during wet grinding:

Increased mill capacity
Lower energy consumption
Elimination of hazards from dust
Easier materials handling

The principal disadvantage, apart from the possible inclusion of a drying stage, is the increased wear of the grinding medium.

## 11.4.2 Contamination

Wear of grinding elements, which occurs in all mills, contaminates the product. Contamination influences the choice of constructional materials, with ceramics and stainless steel most commonly used. Contamination is normally slight. However, in the protracted periods often associated with the production of very fine powders, it may become severe. This is illustrated in Figure 11.2, which shows a progressive increase in a sulfated ash value of the material due to wear of the ceramic mill.

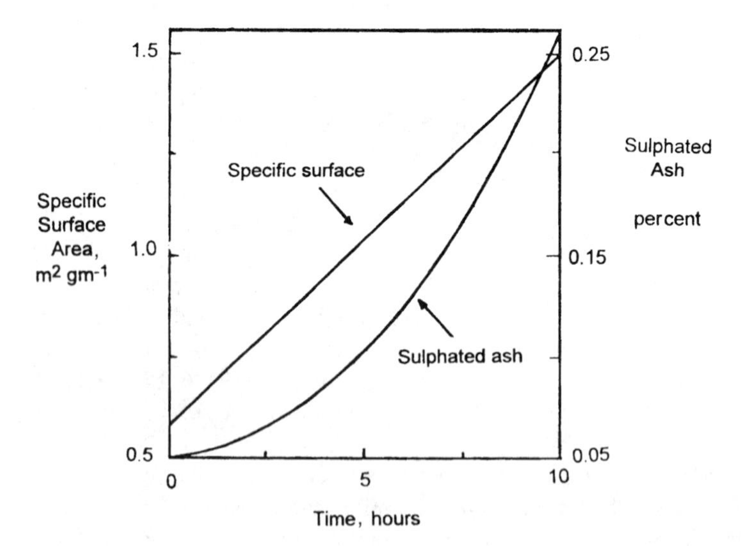


**FIGURE 11.2** Contamination of griseofulvin during milling.

Closed mills, which prevent the ingress of bacteria, must be used for grinding sterile materials.

### 11.4.3 Temperature Sensitivity

Care must be exercised during milling of temperature-sensitive materials, especially when a very fine product is required. Caking results if the softening point is exceeded. Materials may be chilled before grinding, or facilities for cooling the mill during grinding may be provided. Waxy solids can be successfully ground with dry ice, the low temperatures conferring brittle characteristics on the material. Chemical degradation may occur at high grinding temperatures. Oxidative changes can be prevented by grinding in an inert atmosphere such as nitrogen.

### 11.4.4 Structural Changes

Several examples of change of physical structure during very fine grinding have been reported. Gammage and Glasson (1963) found changes in the crystal form of calcium carbonate after ball milling. Distortion of the kaolinite lattice during very fine grinding was reported by Gregg (1955). Changes such as these could affect solubility and other physical characteristics which, in turn, might influence formulation and therapeutic value.

### 11.4.5 Dust Hazards

Hazards from dust may become acute during dry grinding. Extremely potent materials require machines to be dustproof and dustproof clothing and masks to be given to operators. Danger may also arise from the explosive nature of many dusts.

## 11.5 GRINDING EQUIPMENT

The following equipment is in regular use for dry-grinding pharmaceutical materials: edge and end runner mills, hammer mill, pin mills, ball mills.

The fluid energy mill is becoming widely used for producing superfine powders. The ball mill and the colloid mill are used for wet grinding and the production of liquid dispersions. The end runner mill and adaptations of the roll mill may be used to comminute and disperse powders in semisolid bases as, for example, in the production of ointments. These mills, and the vibratory mill, are described in this section.

### 11.5.1 Edge and End Runner Mills

The edge runner mill consists of one or two heavy granite or cast iron wheels or mullers mounted on a horizontal shaft and standing in a heavy pan. Either the muller or the pan is driven. The material is fed into the center of the pan and is worked outward by the muller action. While in the zone traversed by the muller, comminution will occur by compression, due to the weight of the muller, and by shear. The origin of the shear forces is indicated in Figure 11.3(a). The linear velocity of the pan surface will vary over the line of contact between muller and pan. For efficient grinding this dimension is large compared with the diameter of the pan. Muller and pan speeds may only coincide on one hypothetical circle, at other positions a varying amount of slip must occur. A scarper continually moves material from the perimeter of the pan to the grinding zone.

The end runner mill is similar in principle and consists of a rotating pan or mortar made of cast iron or porcelain. A heavy pestle is mounted vertically within the pan in an off-center position [Figure 11.3(b)]. The mechanism of size reduction is compression due to the weight of the pestle, and shear. The latter is developed by the relative movement of muller and pan which varies over the muller face. The muller is friction-driven by the pan through the ground material. A scraper is used to redirect the material into the grinding zone.

Both mills operate at slow speeds on a packed bed. Both produce moderately fine powders and operate successfully with fibrous materials. Wet grinding with very viscous materials, such as ointments and pastes, is also possible.

### 11.5.2 The Hammer Mill

The hammer mill typifies a group of machines operating at very high speeds and acting primarily by impact on a freely suspended particle. The term *disintegrator* is also used. High efficiency, which would be expected from the operation of a free-crushing mechanism, is reduced because the blows delivered are in excess of the minimum required for breakage.

A typical machine [Figure 11.4(a)] consists of a disk rotating at speeds up to 8000 rpm. The higher speeds are used for fine grinding in relatively

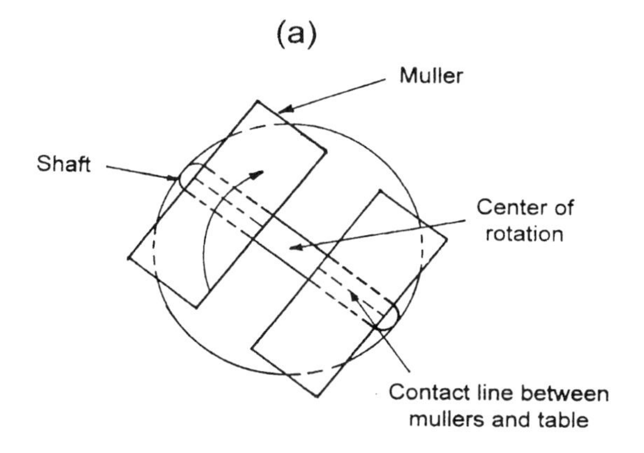


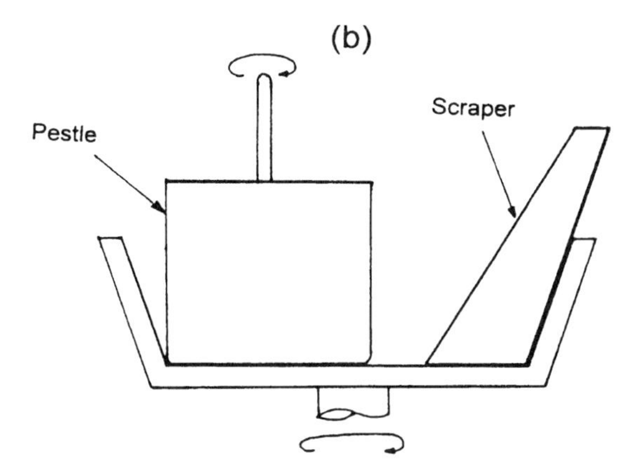


**FIGURE 11.3** (a) Edge runner mill; (b) end runner mill.

small machines. A balanced number of hammers is fitted to the disk. The hammers may be fixed or pivoted, presenting flat, knife, or file edges to the material. The material is fed to the top or the center of the mill and is broken by direct impact until fine enough to pass through the screen which forms the lower part of the mill casing. A range of screens is normally provided. Due to tangential exit, the product size is considerably smaller than the screen apertures. The disk and hammers act as a centrifugal fan, drawing large volumes of air through the mill. Entrained dust must be separated with a bag filter or a cyclone separator.

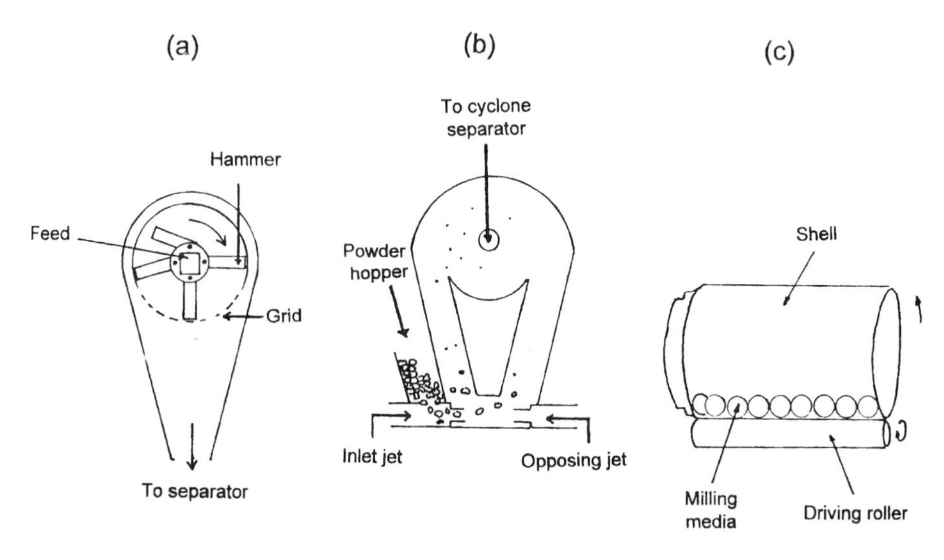


**FIGURE 11.4** (a) Impact mill with pivoted hammers, (b) comminution mill, and (c) ball mill.

The mill processes dry, crystalline materials, which do not soften under milling conditions, and many crude drugs. Rotation speed and size and shape of the screen apertures are interrelated factors controlling the product size. A considerable amount of very fine powder is produced. A marked rise in temperature can occur during passage through the mill with consequent risk of fusion or decomposition of susceptible drugs.

Great versatility, derived from simple variation of screen, rotor speed, and blade type, is characteristic of the refined mills commonly used in the pharmaceutical industry. The Fitzmill (The Fitzpatrick Company of American and Manesty Machines Ltd.) and the Apex Comminuting Mill (Apex Construction Co., London) are mobile machines constructed largely of stainless steel [Figure 11.4(b)]. Both offer a large screen area and operate at various speeds. A reversible rotor permits the use of blades presenting either a flat impact face or a cutting edge to the material. Materials are ground by high-speed operation of the impact face. The knife edges may be used at lower speeds for wet granulation and for precision reduction of the imperfect tablets produced during dry granulation. The mill may be jacketed to control milling temperatures. Mixing, wet grinding, and ointment milling may also be performed.

### 11.5.3 The Pin Mill

Pin mills consist of two horizontal steel plates with vertical projections arranged in concentric circles on opposing faces and becoming more closely spaced toward the periphery. The projections of the two faces intermesh. The material is fed through the center of the stationary upper disk onto the lower revolving disk and is propelled by centrifugal action toward the periphery. The passage between the pins provides size reduction by impact and attrition. The material is collected in the annular space surrounding the disks and passes to a separator. The large volumes of air drawn through the mill are discharged through the separator. Absence of screens and gratings provides clog-free action. The machine is suitable for grinding soft, nonabrasive powders, and low milling temperatures permit heat-sensitive materials to be processed. The fineness of the grind may be varied by the use of disks with different dispositions of pins.

### 11.5.4 The Ball Mill

The ball mill is widely used for fine grinding. Extremely fine powders may be produced, although milling times are often protracted. Despite simple construction, the mill is extremely versatile. It can be used for wet or dry grinding in continuous or batch processes. The latter are usually imposed by the scale of pharmaceutical operations. Since the mill is closed, sterility can be maintained or an operation can be conducted in an inert atmosphere, if the process demands such conditions. Materials of widely differing mechanical properties can be ground by the combined effects of impact and attrition characteristic of the mill.

In its simplest form the ball mill [Figure 11.4(c)] consists of a rotating, hollow cylinder containing balls usually made of stainless steel or stoneware. During grinding, the balls slowly wear and are eventually replaced. For general purposes the mill contains balls of different sizes which perform different functions. Mill loading varies. Typically, it is half-filled with balls, and the material to be ground is added to overfill the interstices between the balls. The apparent volume of the total charge is commonly 60% of the mill volume. In operation the distance the charge moves up the mill casing depends on the centrifugal force, a function of the speed at which the mill rotates and the friction between charge and mill lining. These effects determine the pattern of movement within the mill. At low grinding speeds the balls tumble, roll, and jump down the free face of the charge, a pattern described as *cascading*. With increased speed, the pattern progressively changes to *cataracting* in which the balls are carried almost to the top of the mill and fall directly onto the charge below.

The grinding contributions of impact and attrition vary in these patterns of movement. Attrition predominates in the cascading mill and depends to some extent on the surface area of the balls. The effect can therefore be enhanced by using small balls. Impact breaking becomes more important in the cataracting mill, the most effective action being derived from the high kinetic energy of the larger balls, a factor also influenced by the latter's density.

If there is sufficient friction between the mill lining and the charge, the latter "keys" to the mill at higher speeds and rotates with it. This is termed *centrifuging*, and since there is no relative movement between the balls, no grinding occurs. The speed marking the onset of centrifuging is called the critical speed. Theoretically it represents conditions for which the centrifugal and gravitational forces acting on a ball at the top of the mill are balanced. If the mass of the ball is $m$, the gravitational force is given by $mg$ and the centrifugal force is $mv_c^2/r$, where $v_c$ is the critical speed and $r$ is the distance of the ball from the axis of the mill, i.e., the radius of the mill minus the radius of the ball. These may be equated to give

$$v_c = \sqrt{gr} \tag{11.4}$$

In practice, centrifuging does not occur until well above the theoretical critical speed, and it varies with mill loading and the amount of slip between charge and lining. Mills usually operate at between 50% and 80% of the critical speed. The lower speeds are used for wet grinding and very fine dry grinding.

If a low coefficient of friction permits extensive slipping between mill and charge, centrifuging will not occur even at very high mill speeds. Under these "supercritical" conditions the grinding action differs from the pattern described.

By correct choice of ball size, mill speed, and diameter, the ball mill may be used to grind material of widely different particle size. In coarse dry grinding, the energy associated with the largest ball falling the diameter of the mill must be sufficient to break the largest particle. Very fine grinding, on the other hand, is best effected by the attrition between a large number of small balls. The most important limiting factor in the production of very fine particles by milling is agglomeration. Ultimately, the reduction of new surface by rebonding may equal the increase in surface due to fracture. This is shown

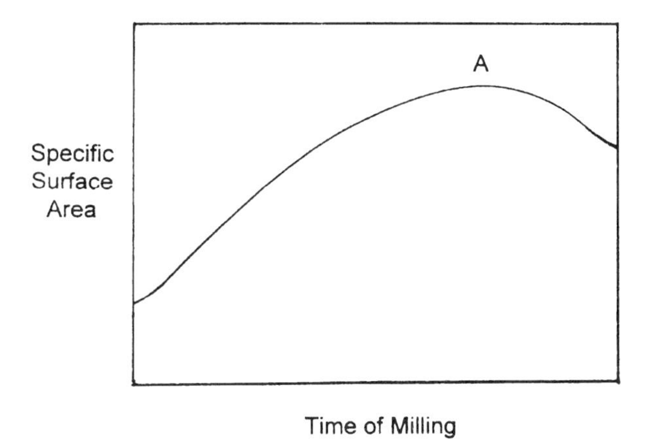


**FIGURE 11.5** Effect of particle agglomeration during milling.

as point A in the relation of specific surface area and milling time in Figure 11.5. With further grinding the effective particle size may actually increase. Agglomeration during fine dry grinding is usually more severe than in wet grinding. In both cases, however, additives can sometimes be used to limit its effect.

The ball mill also provides a simple mechanical means of dispersing solids in liquids. Wet grinding depends on the attrition characteristic of the cascading mill: the smaller the balls the greater the effect, and the greater the suspension viscosity. The latter should not prevent the correct movement of the charge. Where their use is permissible, the addition of surface-active agents may greatly accelerate the process by preventing reaggregation of the particles. Surface-active agents can also alter the physical properties of the solid, lowering the breaking strain and rendering the particle more brittle. A higher ratio of solids to liquid, which aids efficient milling, is possible if the system is deflocculated.

In large-scale, continuous installations, the mill may be modified to apply grinding forces appropriate to the size of particle being ground. In the tube mill the ratio of length to diameter is greatly increased, and the mill is divided into several compartments, each containing balls of different average size. The coarse material first enters the compartment containing the largest balls. It is then conveyed to successive compartments containing smaller balls and capable of progressively finer grinding. In the Hardinge conical ball mill, natural segregation is induced by the conical shape. The largest balls operate at the largest diameter and, through the kinetic energy acquired during the extensive fall, create high-impact stresses suitable for breaking coarse particles. The material first passes through this region. With further progress through the mill, the greater surface presented by the smaller balls promotes finer grinding by attrition.

### 11.5.4 The Vibratory Mill

In the ball mill the grinding energy is derived from the acceleration of the balls in a gravitational field. Under normal conditions the latter limits the speed at which a mill of a given diameter can be run and therefore limits the rate at which energy can be applied to the process. Long milling times are characteristic of the ball mill. The advantage of vibratory milling is centered mainly on this limitation, since it is possible by this method to develop accelerations much greater than those induced by the earth's gravitational field. Grinding can be more energetic and milling times can be greatly reduced.

A simple form of vibratory mill consists of a mill body containing the grinding media, usually of porcelain or stainless steel balls. The mill body is supported on springs which permit an oscillatory movement. This vibration is usually, but not necessarily, in a vertical plane. The suspended mass is maintained in a state of forced vibration by some means, such as the rotation of a shaft on which unbalanced weights are mounted. The charge is subjected to movements of high frequency and small amplitude. The resultant chattering of the mill gives comminution by attrition. Characterized by relatively high speed grinding, the vibratory mill is usually more flexible than the ball mill; charging and discharging and adaption to continuous processing are much easier. The more efficient use of the energy applied and the shorter grinding times usually result in lower milling temperatures than are found in a ball mill. Construction, however, is more complex and the feed size of the material is limited to approximately 0.25 in. and less. The mill is not suitable for grinding resilient materials which cannot be ground by impact since the shear forces developed are less than those found in a ball mill.

A refined example of this principle is found in the Podmore-Boulton Vibro-Energy Mill [Figure 11.6(a)]. This mill consists of an annular grinding chamber generally accommodating a medium of small cylinders. These cylinders align coaxially in a three-dimensional vibratory field to give close packing and line contact between moving surfaces. This alignment, it is claimed, gives

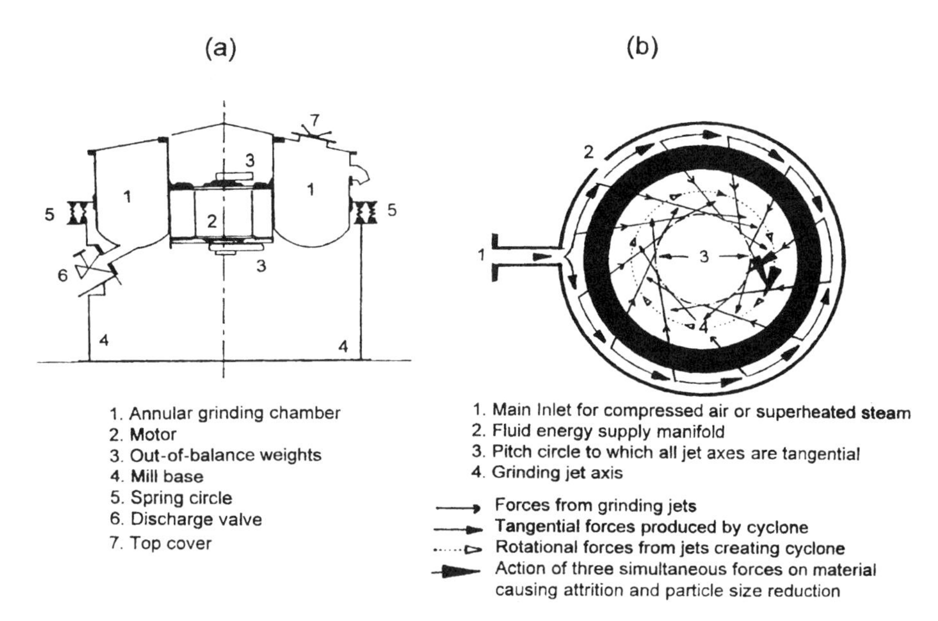


**FIGURE 11.6** (a) Vibro-energy mill and (b) fluid energy mill.

preferential grinding of coarse material leading to products with narrow particle size distributions.

## 11.5.5 The Fluid Energy Mill

The fluid energy mill offers an alternative method of producing very fine powders. The term *micronizer* is in general use and is a trade name coined by a company which originated a particular type of fluid energy mill. In all fluid energy mills the grinding results mainly from attrition between the particles being ground, the energy inducing movement of the particles being supplied in the form of compressed fluids. Air and steam are widely used.

A common type of fluid energy mill is illustrated in Figure 11.6(b). The material is blown into the grinding chamber through a venturi feed placed at its perimeter. The compressed fluid enters the chamber through nozzles tangential to a hypothetical circle within the grinding chamber. The particles are violently accelerated by the rotating fluids and are subjected to the influence of successive nozzles. Grinding results from impact between particles, which are then subjected to the intense classifying action of the circulating fluid. Oversize particles remain in the grinding zone, while fine powder and spent grinding fluid spiral to the central outlet.

For a given machine size reduction depends on the size of the feed, its rate of introduction to the grinding chamber, and the pressure of the grinding fluid. The most important machine factors are the grinding chamber geometry and the number and angle of the nozzles.

Powders with all particles below a few microns may be quickly produced by this method. The disadvantage of high capital and running costs may not be so serious in the pharmaceutical industry because of the high value of the materials which are often processed. For grinding drugs the mill is usually made of stainless steel. Large volumes of air compressed to about $6.89 \times 10^5$ $N/m^2$ must be provided.

### 11.5.6 Colloid Mills

Colloid mills are a group of machines used for wet grinding and dispersion. They operate by shearing relatively thin layers of material between two surfaces, one of which is moving at a high angular velocity relative to the other. Although very fine dispersions can be produced, they are not, as the name implies, of colloidal dimensions. Colloid mills are also widely used to prepare emulsions.

A typical colloid mill consists of a stator and rotor with flat working surfaces, often made of stainless steel or carborundum. The clearance is adjustable from virtually zero upward. The rotor is rotated at several thousand revolutions per minute, and the slurry of already fine material passes through the clearance under the action of centrifugal forces. Surface-active agents fulfill the same function in colloid mills as in ball milling.

### 11.5.7 Roller Mills

Roller mills may be used to grind pastes and other plastic dispersions. They operate by inducing crushing and shearing forces in a thin layer of the paste as it passes through the narrow clearance between two rollers. Commonly, shear forces are intensified by the differing peripheral velocities of the rolls. The clearance between the rolls is variable and depends on the plasticity of the mass, the gap increasing as the stiffness of the material increases. With thin pastes the milling action is similar to that of the colloid mill.

## 11.6 CLASSIFICATION OR SIZE SEPARATION

In the chapter introduction the influence of particle size on several processes was described. The operation in which particles of a suitable size are selected and others rejected because they are too small or too large is called *classification* or *size separation*. This process is also important in closed-circuit grinding, when removing fine powders to promote flow, and when restricting particle size distribution to prevent segregation or to enhance appearance.

Although various particle properties can be used to classify a powder, only two are important. The first is based on the ability of a particle to pass through an aperture, known as *sieving* or *screening*. The second employs the drag forces on a particle moving through a fluid. The term *classification* is sometimes restricted to this method of separation, but in this text *elutriation* and *sedimentation* are used. In general, screening is applied to the separation of coarse particles and elutriation and sedimentation to fine particles.

### 11.6.1 Sieving and Screening

Sieves and screens are widely used in the classification of relatively coarse materials. For very large particles, greater than a half-inch, a robust plate perforated with holes is used. However, the pharmaceutical applications of screening are with much smaller particles, and screens are in the form of woven meshes. Unless special methods are used to prevent clogging and powder aggregation, the lower useful limit resides in a cloth woven with 7900 meshes per meter, corresponding to a mesh spacing between $7.0 \times 10^{-5}$ and $8.0 \times 10^{-5}$ microns. Fine screens of this type are extremely fragile and must be used with great care.

A series of suitable sieve cloths are specified by the gauge of the wire and the permitted weaving tolerances. In successive meshes of this series, the mesh space alters by the factor $4\sqrt{2}$. In the mesh series commonly chosen for size analysis,

16–22–30–44–60–85–120–170

alternate screens are selected so that the mesh spacing decreases by $\sqrt{2}$ and the area of the apertures is halved. For classification one or more meshes of suitable weave can be chosen from this series and mounted in a frame.

In operation the mesh should be lightly loaded so that all particles capable of passing the mesh (undersize) have a chance to do so. The mesh must, therefore, be agitated to ensure access of particles to the holes and to clear holes blocked by particles just unable to pass. Under these conditions the rate of sieving is proportional to the number of undersize particles on the screen. It therefore decreases exponentially.

Most screening, particularly of coarse materials, is carried out dry. Wet screening of dilute slurries is adopted for powders which aggregate strongly, clog the mesh, or become electrostatically charged by the screen vibrations. Sieving errors arising from the cohesion of small and large particles and the retention of the former on a coarse mesh is avoided. Wet screening is particularly useful if the subsequent process is wet and drying is unnecessary.

For small-scale classification, test sieves with meshes mounted on circular brass frames, 8, 12, or 18 in. in diameter, rims on the lower edges enabling them to nest with the sieve beneath. When the chosen sieves are equipped with a lid and receiving pan, the agitated assembly becomes an effective small-scale grading unit. Sieving is stopped when the rate at which particles pass the mesh has reached some low value or after some predetermined time at which the rate is known to be low.

Generally as the scale of the operation increases it becomes less precise. For continuous screening, the feed material is made to move across the screen to a point of discharge. The residence time on the screen is usually short, and many undersize particles traverse it without falling through. With increased sieving area the meshes become more fragile, and the finest meshes must be supported with a coarser wire. An example of a large-scale separator utilizes a circular screen, up to 5 ft in diameter, and vibrates in a horizontal plane, the gyratory movement being imparted by an out-of-balance flywheel connected to the assembly. In other machines the mesh is rectangular and inclined at a shallow angle (5–30°). A gyratory movement is developed and the material to be classified is fed to the top end. These machines may bear more than one deck, thus allowing the powder to be separated into several fractions at one time.

### 11.6.2 Elutriation and Sedimentation

The balance of the drag force on the particle and the forces promoting movement occurs at the terminal velocity. This velocity depends, among other things, on the particle size, and it is the property on which several classifiers are based. The fluid is air or liquid. Liquid affords a higher precision because dispersion can be more thorough. High shear forces cannot be developed, and dispersing agents cannot be used in air.

The simplest classifier is a rising current of fluid in which the particles are suspended. In this case the force opposing the upward drag is gravitational. If the opposition gives a terminal velocity greater than the current speed, the particle will fall. This is the principle of elutriation, and the particle size, *d*, at which the separation is made follows from a rearrangement of equation 1.24 for conditions in which Stokes' law is valid:

$$d = \sqrt{\frac{18\eta u}{(\rho_p - \rho)g}} \tag{11.5}$$

Here $\rho_p - \rho$ is the density difference between solid and fluid, $\eta$ is the viscosity of the fluid, and $u$ is the speed of the upward current.

The elutriator in Figure 11.7(a) consists of three tubes. The first is smallest in diameter and offers the highest upward liquid velocity. Coarse particles with a high terminal velocity settle in this tube while the remainder are swept to the bottom of the second. The diameter of the second tube exceeds that of the first and elutriation speeds are lower. Only fine particles are swept into the third tube, where the process is repeated at a finer size. In this way the original slurry is divided into four fractions.

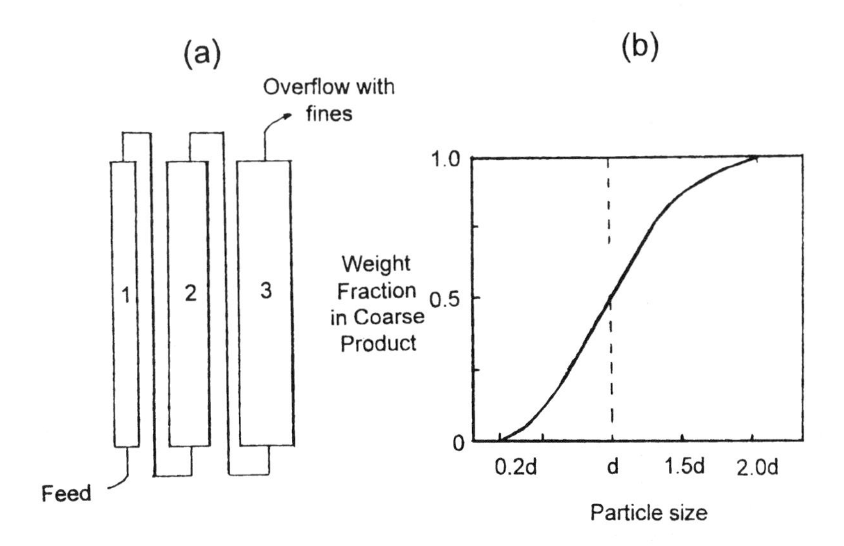


**FIGURE 11.7** (a) Elutriator and (b) grade efficiency curve.

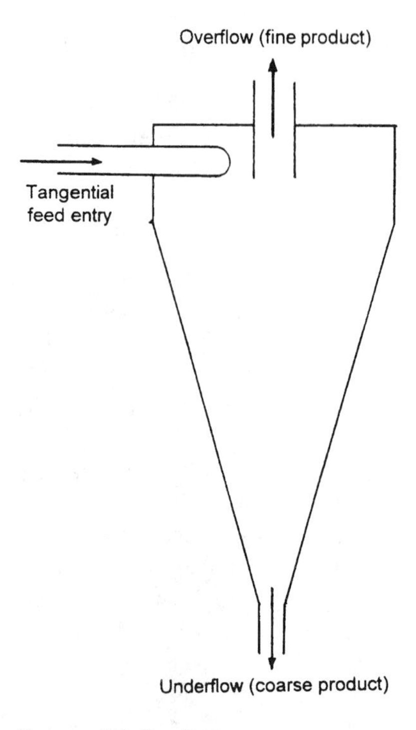


**FIGURE 11.8** Cyclone separator.

In practice, fluctuations in flow conditions due to natural convection and a violation of the conditions for which Stokes' law is valid blur the point of separation. Evaluating the separation must, therefore, take account of the fine particles which fall with the coarse particles and of the coarse particles which move to the fine fraction. This is best expressed by a grade efficiency curve. Returning to equation 1.24, a particle of size $d$ should be stationary in the elutriation tube. Due to fluctuating conditions it eventually resides with the coarse or fine fractions, the chances being equal. The weight fraction in each is, therefore, 0.5 at this size. We shall assume that of the particles which are twice this size ($2d$), virtually all appear in the coarse product.

The weight fraction here is unity. Similarly, all particles of size $0.2d$ move to the fine product, so the weight fraction in the coarse product is zero. As shown in Figure 11.7(b), a sigmoid curve, passing through 0.5 at size $d$, links these extremes. The closer these extremes and the steeper the curve, the more efficient is the separation. A grade efficiency curve of this type can be used as an appraisal of any sedimentor or elutriator.

Gravitational sedimentation is not of great importance in small-scale classification. Sedimentation in a spinning fluid stream is, however, widely used. The most common classifier of this type is the cyclone separator in Figure 11.8. The fluid enters tangentially and acquires an intense spinning motion, spiraling downward into the cone before rising to the outlet as a central core. The inlet speed is very high, so large angular velocities are developed. Due to centrifugal force particles move radially across the spinning stream to fall at the wall into the cone. Operated in this way complete separation of solids occurs and the cyclone is, therefore, an effective air cleaner. Operated with lower centrifugal forces the cyclone transports the finest particles to the exhaust, leaving the coarser particles to fall into the cone. Cyclone classifiers are designed for use with liquid or air.

The centrifuge is normally operated to completely separate two phases. If, however, the rate at which the feed passes through does not allow all particles to settle, the action of a classifier is developed. This is illustrated by a solid bowl centrifuge which consists of a steel shell in the form of a frustum mounted horizontally. It contains a conveying screw at the wall which rotates at a slightly higher speed than the shell. Particles which settle at the wall are conveyed to the narrow end of the shell and discharged. Fine particles are entrained with the overflow to the other end.

# 12

# Mixing

## 12.1 INTRODUCTION

Perry and Chilton (1973) defined mixing as an operation "in which two or more ingredients in separate or roughly mixed condition are treated so that each particle of any one ingredient is as nearly as possible adjacent to a particle of each of the other ingredients." The term *blending* is synonymous with mixing, and *segregation* or *demixing* is the opposite. Mixing is a basic step in most process sequences, and it is normally carried out

1. To secure uniformity of composition so that small samples withdrawn from a bulk material represent the overall composition of the mixture
2. To promote physical or chemical reactions, such as dissolution, in which natural diffusion is supplemented by agitation

Mixing can be classified as positive, negative, or neutral. *Positive mixing*, which applies to systems that, given time, would spontaneously and completely mix, such as two gases or two miscible liquids. Mixing apparatus is used on such systems to accelerate mixing. *Negative mixing* is demonstrated by suspensions of solids in liquids. Any two-phase system, in which the phases differ in density, will separate unless continuously agitated. *Neutral mixing* occurs when neither mixing nor demixing takes place unless the system is acted on by a system of forces. Examples are mixing solids with solids and solids with liquids when the solids concentration is high.

Mixing must embrace all combinations of the three states of matter. The theory of mixing should be able, when the system to be mixed has been defined, to dictate the type and design of the mixer, such as volume, shape, and type of impeller, and the process conditions, such as degree of agitation and the time and power required. Theoretical knowledge is, however, insufficient to predict mixer performance. More commonly, choice is based on broad empirical principles which are then supported by practical tests.

## 12.2 THE SCALE OF SCRUTINY

Whether materials are satisfactorily mixed depends on the subsequent operations in which the mixture plays a part. Any mixture, if examined on a small enough scale, shows regions of segregation. An acceptable degree of mixing is related to subsequent operations in a process sequence. The term *scale of scrutiny* is used to describe the minimum size of the regions of segregation in a mixture which would cause it to be regarded as insufficiently mixed. For example, if a tablet is to contain 0.1 g of drug A and 0.1 g of drug B, the powder from which the tablets are to be made must be sufficiently mixed so that, on drawing a sample of 0.2 g from the mixture, the sample contains, within narrow limits, the correct amounts of A and B. The way in which A and B are dispersed within the sample may be of no importance as long as the tablet is not divided. The scale of scrutiny is here determined by the tablet weight. In general, a small scale of scrutiny is applied if the unit size of the product is small and if too much or too little of one component is very undesirable.

Two further useful concepts to describe unmixedness are the scale of segregation and the intensity of segregation. The *scale of segregation* is a measure of the size of the regions of unmixed materials. In the preceding example the intensity of segregation shows the extent to which A has been diluted with B, and vice versa. These two concepts are usually interrelated. A high *intensity of segregation* can be tolerated as long as the scale of segregation is small. Alternatively, a larger scale of segregation may be tolerated if the intensity of segregation is reduced.

## 12.3 MIXING OF SOLIDS

Pharmacy offers many important examples of mixing solids. In several forms of drug presentation, the attainment of accurate dosage depends on an adequate mixing operation at some stage in production. Since the dose unit may be small, say 0.1 g, a small scale of scrutiny is applied.

The mixing of all systems of matter involves a relative displacement of the particles—whether molecules, globules, or small crystals—until a state of maximum disorder is created and a completely random arrangement is achieved. Such an arrangement for a mixture of equal parts of two components is shown in Figure 12.1(b).

A ''perfect'' mixture, which, with a practical sample, would offer point uniformity, is shown in Figure 12.1(a). Such an arrangement is, however, virtually impossible, and no mixing equipment can do better than produce the ''random'' mixture in Figure 12.1(b). In such a mixture the probability of finding one type of particle at any point in the mixture is equal to the proportion of that type of particle in the mixture.

Mixing solids differs from mixing liquids in that the smallest practical sample withdrawn from a mixture of two miscible liquids contains many millions of particles. In solids mixing a small sample contains relatively few particles, and examination of Figure 12.1(b) should show that such samples exhibit

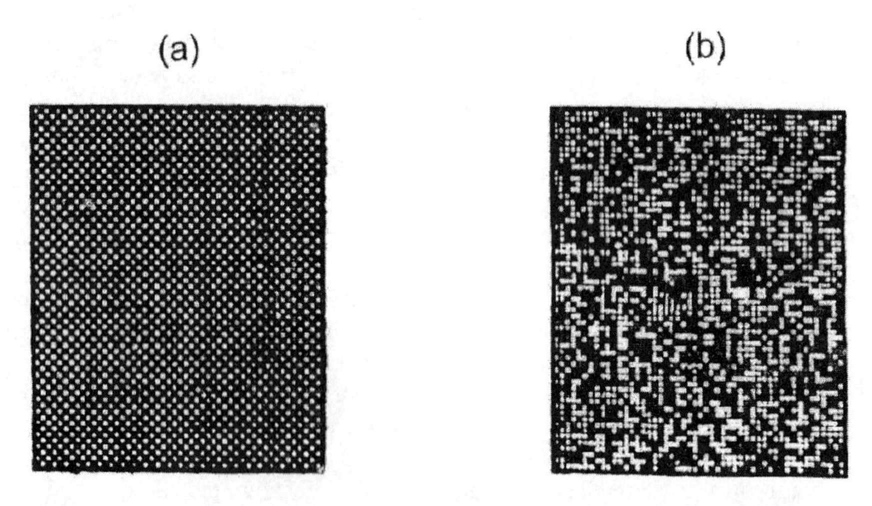


**FIGURE 12.1** Diagrammatic representation of (a) a perfect mix and (b) a random mix.

considerable variation with respect to the overall mixture composition and that this variation should be reduced as the number of particles in the sample increases. Assessing the variation in, say, drug content in a series of samples drawn from a mixture of powders is of great importance. The tablet machine may be regarded as a volumetric sampling device, and the variation in drug content between one tablet and the next is largely controlled by the mixing stage which precedes it.

### 12.3.1 Some Properties of a Random Mixture

In 1943, Lacey (1953) showed that the variation in the composition of samples drawn from a random mixture of two materials could be expressed by the relation

$$s = \sqrt{\frac{p(1 - p)}{n}} \tag{12.1}$$

where $s$ is the standard deviation of the samples, $p$ is the proportion of one component, and $n$ is the number of particles in the sample. The relation requires that the two components be alike in particle size, shape, and density and only be distinguished by some neutral property, such as color. If a very large number of samples, each containing a given number of particles, is withdrawn from a mixture of equal parts of two materials, the results of analysis can be presented in the form of a frequency curve in which the samples are normally distributed around the mean content of the mixture. A total of 99.7% of the samples will fall within the limits $p = 0.5 + 3\sigma$. The standard deviation of the samples is inversely proportional to the square root of the number of particles in a sample. If the particle size is reduced so that the same weight of sample contains four times as many particles, the standard deviation is halved. The distribution of samples and the effect of size reduction are shown in Figure 12.2.

In a critical examination of pharmaceutical mixing, Train showed that samples of a random mixture of equal parts of A and B must contain at least 800 particles if 997 out of every 1000 samples ($3\sigma$) were to lie between $\pm 10\%$ of the stated composition; i.e., the proportion, $p$, of A $= 0.5 \pm 0.05$, whence $\sigma = 0.05/3$ (Train, 1960). The effect of the number of particles in a sample on the percentage variation about the mean content of a mixture of equal parts A and B was summarized by Train [Figure 12.3]. The diagram may be used to show that if, in the example, limits of $\pm 1\%$ were substituted, 90,000 particles must be present in each sample. The true standard deviation is symbolized

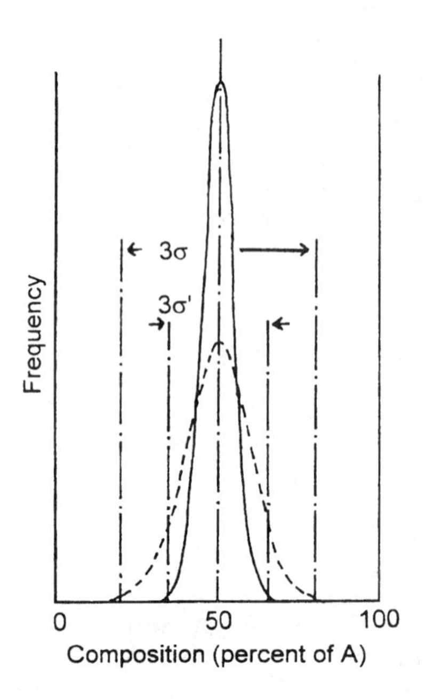


**FIGURE 12.2** Distribution of samples drawn from a mixture of equal parts A and B. The broken line represents data for the coarser powder.

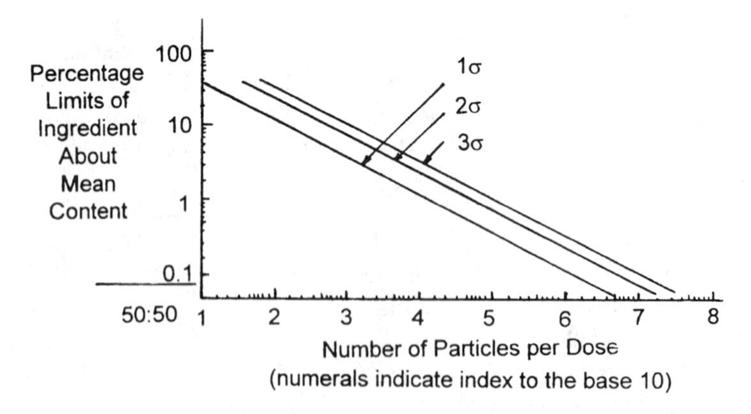


**FIGURE 12.3** General theoretical relationship between number of particles and percentage limit of ingredient for a 50:50 mix.

by $\sigma$. The standard deviation estimated by the withdrawal of a number of samples is denoted by $s$.

If instead of equal parts A and B, the proportion of an active ingredient, A, in the mixture were 0.1 (10%), imposition of limits of $\pm 10\%$ (in 997 cases out of 1000) requires that each sample contain over 8000 particles. If the proportion of active constituent is 0.01 or 1%, a figure of 90,000 particles per sample is obtained, and if the limits are reduced to $\pm 1\%$, the figure is 9 million.

The theoretical derivation of these results is based on component particles which are alike in size, shape, and density. This condition is not encountered in the practical mixing of solids, and, as we shall see, any of these factors may prevent the formation of a random mixture. The value of the number of particles per sample derived in any example must therefore be raised if the limits given are to be maintained.

As the proportion of an active ingredient in a mixture decreases, the number of particles in each sample or dose must increase and materials of smaller particle size must be used. This statement indicates the limitation of the mixing of solids. Producing very fine powders is difficult and often attended by severe aggregation, thus defeating the object of size reduction in the mixing process. Where the proportion of active constituent is very small and is finally presented in a small-dose unit, dry mixing of solids may fail to produce an adequate dispersion of one component in another, and other methods, such as spraying a solution of one component onto another, must then be adopted.

Another example of the relation of dose uniformity and number of particles in the dose is two components which are separately granulated before mixing. This procedure is sometimes adopted for reasons of stability during granulation. The variation in samples drawn from such a system is much greater than the variations in a mixture which was mixed before granulation, because the effective number of particles in the sample is greatly reduced.

### 12.3.2 Degree of Mixing

A quantitative expression which defines the state of a mix is necessary if a rational answer to the question, Is this material well enough mixed? is to be made. Such an expression would also allow the course of mixing to be followed and the performances of different mixers to be compared. The most useful way to express the degree of mixing is to measure the statistical variation in composition of a number of samples drawn from the mix. The scale of scrutiny determines the size of the sample, and their number depends on the accuracy required of the assessment.

As already shown, a series of samples drawn from a random mix exhibits a standard deviation of $s_r$. An index of mixing, $M$, is given by

$$M = \frac{s_r}{s} \tag{12.2}$$

where $s$ is the standard deviation of samples drawn from the mixture under examination. This approaches unity as mixing is completed:

$$M' = \frac{s_0 - s}{s_0^2 - s_r} \tag{12.3}$$

where $s_0$ is the standard deviation of samples drawn from the unmixed materials. It is equal to $p(1 - p)$, where $p$ is the proportion of the component in the mix. Its modification by Lacey, using the variance of the samples, to

$$M'' = \frac{s^2 - s_r^2}{s_0^2 - s_r^2} \tag{12.4}$$

gives a fundamental equation for expressing the state of the mixture, where $M''$ varies from zero to unity.

The binomial and Poisson distributions have also been used to examine the state of a mixture. If the proportion of black particles in a random mixture of black and white particles is $p$, the probability, $P(x)$, of obtaining $x$ black particles in a sample of $n$ particles is

$$P(x) = \binom{n}{x} p^x (1 - p)^{n-x} \tag{12.5}$$

If $p$ is small ($<0.15$) and $n$ is large, the Poisson distribution can be used when

$$P(x) = e^{-m(m^x/x!)} \tag{12.6}$$

where $m = np$, the mean number of black particles in the samples of $n$ particles. This relation may be used in an assessment of dry mixing equipment.

If $m > 20$ and more than 10 samples are taken, then:

1. About 10 of the samples have the number of black particles outside the limits $m \pm 1.7\sqrt{m}$.
2. About 5% of the samples have the number of black particles outside the limits $m \pm 2.0\sqrt{m}$.
3. About 1% of the samples have the number of black particles outside the limits $m \pm 2.6\sqrt{m}$.

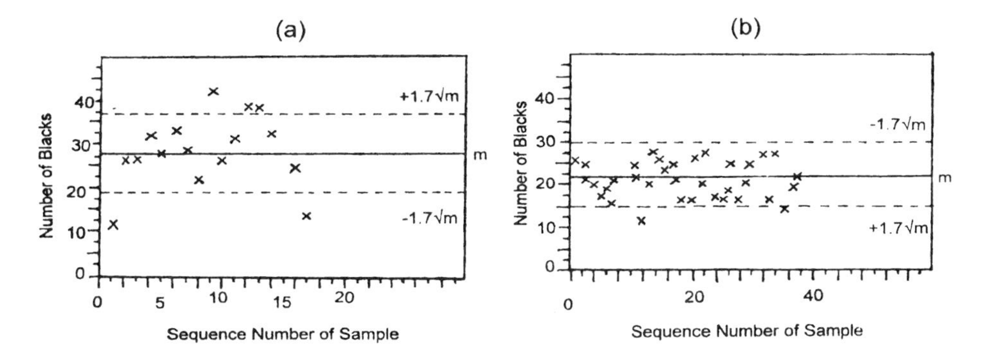


**FIGURE 12.4** Variation in the number of black particles in samples drawn from a tumbler blender for (a) $p < 0.01$ and (b) $p = 0.7$.

Results of such tests in which small cubes of polythene were mixed in a double-cone blender are shown in Figure 12.4(a,b). The probability that the results plotted in Figure 12.4(a) came from a random mixture is less than 0.01, 19 out of 34 samples exceeding the 1 in 10 limits. The densities of the two components in this example were 0.92 and 1.2. The results in Figure 12.4(b) were obtained when the components were of the same density and the probability that the samples were drawn from a random mixture was 0.7.

Alternatively, satisfactory mixing may be established by imposing standards dictated by the operations in which the mixture is to take part. The variance of the samples at different times during mixing is shown in Figure 12.5. The samples, which in this case weighed 5 g, represent the ultimate subdivision of a production size antibiotic mixture. An acceptable degree of homogeneity was set at a standard deviation of 5%, giving a variance of $(0.05)^2$, and this was achieved after just over 100 revolutions of the mixer. [The band around the experimental values of the variance defines the limits within which the true variance lies ($p = 0.9$).] By this method the suitability of the machine and operating characteristics were established.

### 12.3.3 Mechanisms of Mixing and Demixing

The randomization of particles by relative movement, one to another, is achieved by the following mechanisms:

1. *Convective mixing*: transferring groups of adjacent particles from one location in the mass to another

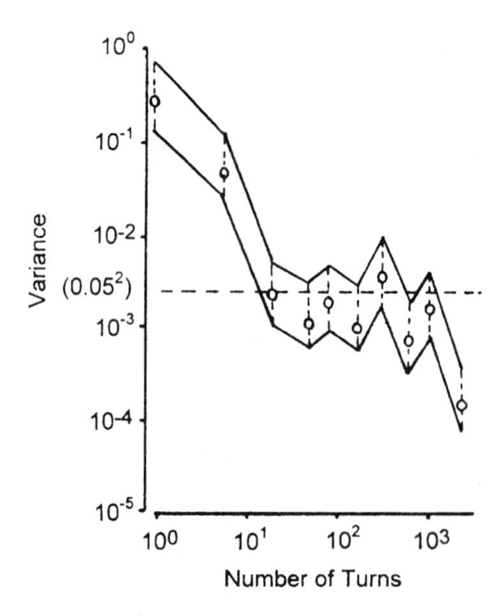


**FIGURE 12.5** Decrease in the variance of samples drawn from a mixture of penicillin (40%) and dihydrostreptomycin in a twin-shell blender.

2. *Diffiusive mixing*: distributing particles over a freshly developing surface
3. *Shear mixing*: setting up slip planes within the mass

All take place to some extent during mixing, but they vary in extent with the type of mixer used. In general, a large diffusional element is necessary if the scale of scrutiny is small. In addition, distortion of portions of the material by intense shear forces, as in mulling, and the scattering of individual particles by impact, processes normally associated with size reduction, are used for some mixing operations.

Convective mixing predominates in machines utilizing a mixing element moving in a stationary container. An example is the horizontal ribbon mixer. Groups of adjacent particles are moved from one position to another, giving a steady decrease in the scale of segregation.

Shear mixing occurs when a system of forces acting on the particles induces the formation of a slip place. This gives relative displacement of two regions. It occurs, for example, in shape rearrangement as the main charge falls from end to end in a double-cone mixer. Train has stressed the importance of expansion or dilation of the material, so shear forces may be effective (Train, 1960). A practical corollary is that efficiency is reduced if the machine is overfilled.

Diffusive mixing predominates in tumbler mixers. Tumbling occurs as the material is lifted past its angle of repose. Mixing occurs when a particle changes its path of circulation through a collision or when it is trapped in voids presented by another layer of particles.

The mild forces involved in these examples may be insufficient to adequately disperse materials which tend to aggregate. The more energetic processes of mulling and impact milling may then be used. Size reduction and mixing are carried out simultaneously, although the former may be slight. An example is the incorporation of ferric oxide and basic zinc carbonate in calamine production. For mixing of this type the hammer mill, mullers, and ball mills charged with small balls are frequently used. The material being processed at any time must contain the correct amounts of materials. If the holdup capacity of the mill is sufficiently large, this can be achieved by a correctly proportioned feed. Otherwise, the product must be mixed a second time by some other method to correct segregation of large-scale but small intensity.

If all particles in a mixture reacted equally to an applied force, then all mixers would eventually produce a random mixture, although the time taken would vary, the more efficient mixer producing a random mix more quickly. The characteristics of real mixtures prevent this, and differences in particle size, shape, and density oppose randomization. Of these, differences in particle size are the most important. The role of these factors in opposing mixing and promoting demixing is demonstrated in the analysis of horizontal drum mixing. Movement of material in a radial plane is shown in Figure 12.6. The static mass of particles is lifted past its angle of repose, and particles tumble down

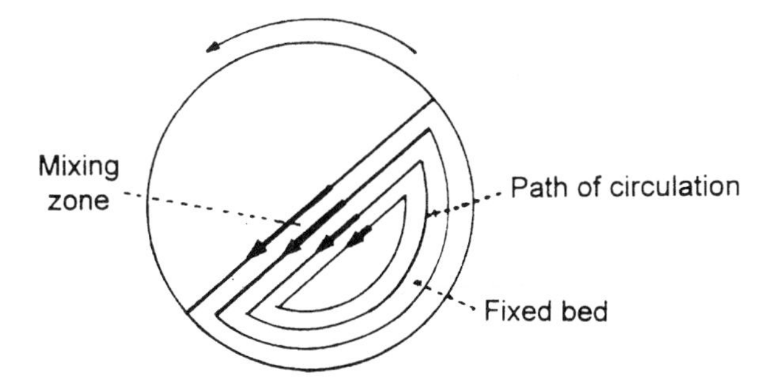


**FIGURE 12.6** Mechanism of radial mixing and demixing.

the free surface, accelerating to the center of the mixer and then decelerating before entering the static bed. The zone in which this takes place is the mixing zone, and since it is in contact with the static bed, in which no mixing takes place and which is moving in the opposite direction, a velocity gradient occurs across the mixing zone; i.e., a layer of particles is passing over the layer beneath, and so on. This zone is in an expanded state and particles are therefore passing over voids in the layer beneath. Mixing occurs when a particle is trapped by moving into a void, thus changing its path of circulation. This mechanism suggests an optimal running speed. If it is too slow, not enough events occur. If it is too fast, the capture time is insufficient.

As long as one type of particle is not preferentially caught, a random mix eventually occurs in the radial plane. If, however, one component is smaller, denser, or has certain shape characteristics, it is preferentially trapped and moves into the lower layers of the mixing zone until it finally concentrates as a central core running the length of the mixer. Similar effects occur in axial mixing, and the final shape of the segregated zone formed under the influence of axial and radial movement depends on the material's flow properties. Similar effects occur with a double-cone blender. Segregation also occurs with such materials when they are dumped from the mixer.

In general, one component concentrates at one position in the mixer when a simple-repetitive, symmetric movement occurs. Modern design tends to the rotation of asymmetric shapes or to symmetric shapes rotated asymmetrically, often with an abrupt reversal in charge movement. Even so, segregation may still occur after a long period of mixing. The variance of samples decreases during mixing to a minimum value, and is followed by a period of demixing, the variance finally achieving a higher equilibrium value. It is therefore possible to overmix.

### 12.3.4 Mixing Rate

Since mixing is a process of achieving uniform randomness, the mixing rate is proportional to the amount of mixing still to be done. If, at the start of mixing, a particle changes its path of circulation, it is most likely to find itself in a different environment. The rate of mixing is therefore fast. At the end of the process, the particle is less likely to find a different environment, and such a change gives no useful mixing. Fewer mixing events take place, and the mixing rate finally reaches zero. The mixing rate for any mixing mechanism can be represented by the expression

$$\frac{dM}{dt} = k(1 - M) \qquad (12.7)$$

where $M$, the mixing index, has already been defined. Integrating this equation gives

$$M = 1 - e^{-kt} \tag{12.8}$$

The rate constant $k$ depends on the physical nature of the materials being mixed and on mixer geometry and operation.

## 12.4 MIXING MACHINES

### 12.4.1 Trough, Ribbon, and Paddle Mixers

A simple trough mixer consists of a semicircular trough in which an impeller, such as paddles mounted at diverse angles on a shaft running the length of the trough, rotates, thereby lifting and distributing the material in an irregular manner. Convective and shear mixing occur. Some fine-scale diffusive mixing occurs when the impeller lifts material clear of the main charge.

The ribbon mixer employs a ribbon-like conveying scroll. The helix, which may be continuous or interrupted, is rotated in a semicircular trough, and mixing again occurs through convection and shear, giving rapid coarse-scale dispersion. Two ribbons set to convey material in opposite directions are frequently fitted to the shaft. Although little axial mixing in the vicinity of the shaft occurs, mixtures with high homogeneity can be produced by prolonged mixing even when components differ in particle size, shape, or density or there is some tendency to aggregate.

### 12.4.2 Tumbler Mixers

Tumbler mixers operate by a mainly diffusive mechanism, their use is confined to free-flowing and granular materials. The mild forces employed, which preclude mixing materials which aggregate strongly, allows friable materials to be handled satisfactorily. The more elaborate geometric forms are most commonly used because movement of material in all planes, which is necessary for rapid overall mixing, is induced. Internal baffles and lifter blades may also be incorporated. For example, axial movement of material along the length of a simple drum mixer is slow and can be enhanced by these methods.

### 12.4.3 Mullers and Impact Millers

The function of mullers and impact millers was discussed earlier.

## 12.5 MIXING LIQUIDS

In mixing miscible liquids, any practical scale of scrutiny embraces a very large number of particles. If, therefore, a mixture of liquids is randomized by agitation, for all practical purposes it can be regarded as uniform. Miscible liquids are classified as positive mixtures and would, given time, mix completely without external help. The time required for mixing is reduced by agitation during which the scale of segregation is reduced, allowing a fast decay in the intensity of segregation by natural diffusion. In general, no great problems are encountered unless the operational scale is very large.

Miscible liquids are most commonly mixed by impellers rotating in tanks. These impellers are classified as

1. Paddles
2. Propellers
3. Turbines

In conjunction with the design of the containing vessel, impellers provide

a. A region of intense shear near the impeller with the induction of high-velocity gradients and turbulence within the liquid.
b. Projection of the disturbance as a flow pattern extending throughout the volume of the container. This is dictated by the impeller's type and position, the tank design, and the material's flow properties.

All the material should pass through the impeller zone at frequent intervals of time, the design of the mixer preventing the formation of ''dead'' zones. The turbulent, high-velocity flow of liquid from the impeller causes mixing by projecting eddies into, and entraining liquid from, the neighboring zones. The thin ribbons of one component in another rapidly become diffuse and finally disappear through molecular diffusion.

The flow pattern may be analyzed in terms of its three components of motion: *radial flow* (i.e., perpendicular to the impeller shaft); *longitudinal* or *axial flow* (i.e., parallel to the shaft); and *tangential flow* (i.e., a circular path around the shaft). A satisfactory flow pattern depends on the correct balance of these components. In a cylindrical tank, radial flow gives rise to axial flow by reaction at the tank wall. Tangential flow receives no such modification. Its predominance as laminar flow circulation supports stratification at various levels. Furthermore, a vortex is created at the liquid surface which may penetrate to the impeller, causing air to be dispersed in the liquid. In general, tangential flow should be minimized by moving the impeller to an off-center position, thus destroying mixer symmetry, or by modifying the flow pattern with baffles. Tanks with vertical agitators may be baffled by one, two, or more strips mounted vertically on, or just away from, the vessel wall. Baffles reduce, but do not eliminate, tangential flow, whereas little modification of radial and axial flow occurs. Baffles produce additional turbulence.

Additional factors must be applied to mixing two immiscible liquids. This operation, encountered, for example, in liquid-liquid extraction, involves the production and maintenance of a large interfacial contact area. In addition, phase separation due to differences in density must be opposed by an adequate axial flow pattern. The high rates of shear induced by propeller or turbine rotation cause globules of the disperse phase to be drawn into an unstable filament of liquid which breaks and re-forms into smaller globules. Unless stabilized by surface-active agents, the reverse process—coalescence—occurs in zones in which velocity gradients are small.

### 12.5.1 Paddle Mixers

Four types of paddle mixers are illustrated in Figure 12.7. The mixing element is large in relation to the vessel and rotates at low speeds (10–100 rpm). A simple paddle, with upper and lower blades, suitable for mixing miscible liquids of low viscosity is shown in Figure 12.7(a). A tangential flow pattern predominates with zones of turbulence to the rear of the blades. The gate paddle in Figure 12.7(b) is suitable for mixing liquids of higher viscosity, and the anchor paddle in Figure 12.7(d), with low clearance between pan and blade, is useful for working across a heat transfer surface. Stationary paddles intermeshing with the moving element suppress swirling in the mixer in Figure 12.7(c). In the other examples baffles are necessary. Unless paddle blades are pitched, poor axial turnover of the liquid occurs. Hence, paddles are not suitable for mixtures which separate.

### 12.5.2 Propeller Mixers

Propellers are commonly used for mixing miscible and immiscible liquids of low viscosity. The marine propeller is typical of the group. High-speed rotation (400–1500 rpm) of the relatively small element provides high shear rates in the vicinity of the impeller and a flow pattern with mainly axial and tangential components. They may be used in unbaffled tanks when mounted in an off-center position or inclined from the vertical. Horizontal mounting in the side of the vessel is frequently used when the scale of the operation is large.

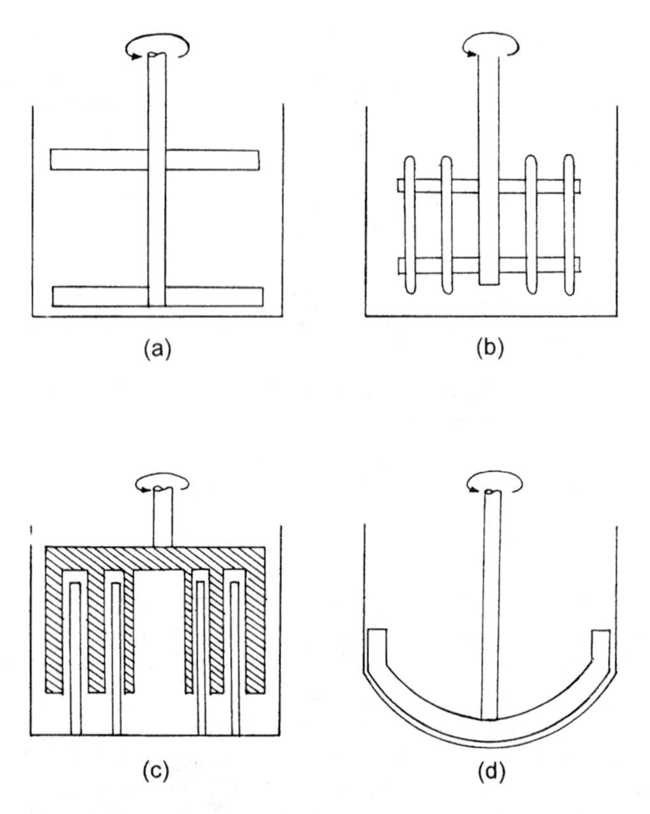


**FIGURE 12.7** Paddle mixers.

## 12.5.3 Turbines

Turbine designs are intermediate between paddles and propellers. Turbines are effective mixers over a wide viscosity range and provide a very versatile mixing tool. The ratio of radial to tangential flow, which are the predominating components with this impeller, increases as the operating speed increases. Pitched-blade turbines are sometimes used to increase axial flow Baffles must be used to limit swirling unless a shrouded turbine is used. With this impeller a discharge with no tangential component is produced.

## 12.5.4 Mixing Liquids and Solids

Examples of solid-liquid mixing occur during dissolution and crystallization and in controlling chemical reactions between solids and liquids. Alternatively randomization of materials for subdivision and presentation may be the object, as, for example, in toothpaste production.

The flow properties of a liquid-solid mixture alter markedly with change in the ratio of the two phases. At low, solid-disperse phase concentrations, flow properties are Newtonian and mixing by impellers is satisfactory as long as flow components oppose settling. Under such conditions it may be desirable to increase impeller size and decrease its speed. For a given power input, improved flow patterns are produced at the expense of turbulence. Unless the difference in density between solid and liquid is small, paddles are ineffective for suspending solids. Otherwise, the discussion presented for mixing liquids may be applied.

Anomalous flow characteristics are exhibited at higher disperse phase concentrations in which the apparent viscosity is a function of the shear rate. The apparent viscosity may increase or, more commonly, decrease as speed impeller increases. Mixing is achieved by suitable impellers, notably the turbine, as long as adequate flow patterns in the entire volume of the mixing vessel are created. Turbulence is less effective as a mixing mechanism, and regimes of laminar flow will be extensive.

Further increase in apparent viscosity occurs at higher disperse phase concentrations. This is often associated with the development of a yield value. Unlike true liquids, shear forces must exceed a certain level before deformation occurs. Since the shear forces developed by particles suspended in liquids are small, sedimentation does not occur and the mixture may be classified as neutral. Mixing by impellers is precluded if the apparent viscosity is very high, because the projection of adequate flow patterns is impossible. Alternative methods must be used in which the mixing element visits all stations in the mixing vessel. For thin pastes, machines typified by the domestic food mixer are used. Imposition of planetary movement on the rotation of the mixing element causes all parts of the mix to be sheared at intervals. Very high shear rates are produced as the element sweeps out zones close to the container wall. In other machines, the containing vessel rotates.

For thicker pastes and plastics, a kneading, stretching, and folding action is employed. The sigma blade, mounted axially in a trough, is a commonly used mixing element. Intense shear is induced by the close clearance between element and container. Simultaneous transport around the trough occurs, so all portions of the mass are periodically deformed. Considerable variation in rheological properties may occur during mixing, and robust mixer construction is essential.

The differential speed of the rolls of the roll mill induces high shear rates in the material. This machine is suitable for paste mixing. With more fluid dispersions, the ball mill and the colloid mill may be used. Solids which aggregate may be successfully dispersed, although subsequent stability may require a deflocculating agent.

Blending solids with very small quantities of liquid, an operation commonly used for granulating powders, presents extreme problems of uniformity. If the material does not become plastic and pasty, it will not mix by shear deformation in the manner described. Mixing is then best achieved by spraying the liquid as fine droplets onto a highly mobile powder which is continually and rapidly developing new surfaces. In this way all particles can be exposed to the spray. A closed ribbon mixer, planetary mixer, or sigma blade mixer can be used. Alternatively, tumbler mixers can be fitted with a spray device. If the solid is itself a mixture, the material must be completely mixed before liquid is added. Otherwise, homogeneity is difficult to achieve.

# 13

# Solid Dosage Forms

Earlier the subject of powders was addressed from a physicochemical standpoint. The unit processes involved in incorporating powders in solid dosage forms must also be considered. Solid dosage forms can be divided into granules, capsules, and tablets for oral delivery, and inhalation products. Note that solid particulates might also play a role in certain parenterals in the form of reconstitutable products.

Solid dosage forms are the most desirable final products of a development process that begins with drug discovery, proceeds through bulk product manufacturing, preformulation, and formulation characterization to one of the products mentioned. Figure 13.1 illustrates an abbreviated sequence of steps through which the drug passes to the final dosage form.

Most solid dosage forms are intended for oral ingestion. The drug released from the dosage form is available at the site of absorption or action within the gastrointestinal tract.

Preformulation studies are required before a formulation is developed. By studying the properties of the drug it is possible to delineate a course of action for composing the formulation. The properties studied are

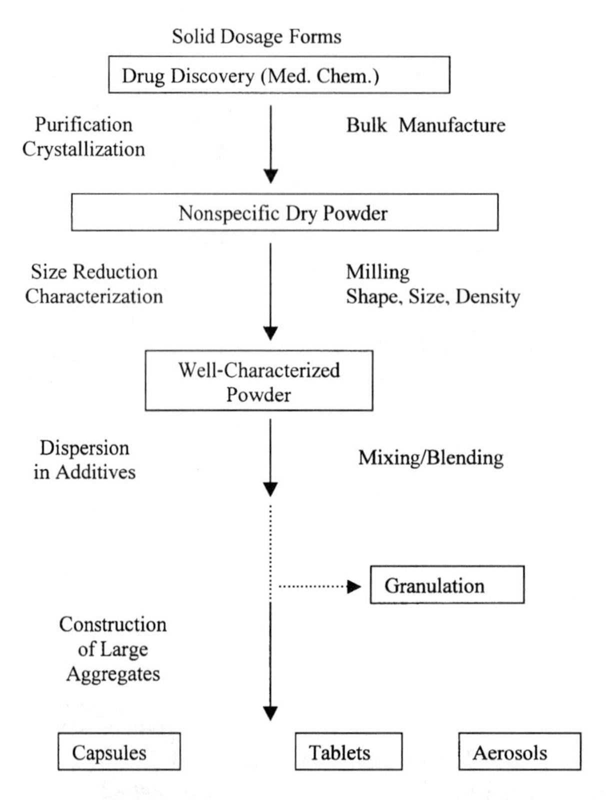


**FIGURE 13.1** Drug to the final dosage form.

- Organoleptic properties
- Purity
- Particle size, shape, and surface area
- Solubility
- Dissolution
- Parameters affecting absorption (dissociation constant, partition coefficient)
- Crystal properties and polymorphism
- Stability (chemical and physical)
- Compatibility (with excipients and potential packaging materials)
- Miscellaneous physicochemical properties
  Density
  Hygroscopicity

Flowability
Compressibility
Wettability

Problem solving in service of formulation development can be derived from knowledge of these properties. Each item has been covered in depth elsewhere and is beyond the scope of this volume.

The additives employed in solid dosage forms are categorized as diluent, glidant, lubricant, disintegrant, and binder. Several candidates from each category may be considered as components of a possible dosage form. Lubricants and disintegrants play a more substantial role in compressed tablet dosage forms than they do in granules or capsules. This will be discussed in more detail later.

## 13.1 GRANULATION

The simplest form of solid dosage form employs granules prepared from the drug and other components in stable aggregates in sizes large enough to facilitate accurate manipulation and dispensing in bulk and at the level of the unit dose.

Following particle size reduction and blending the formulation may be granulated (Carstensen, 1993), which provides homogeneity of drug distribution in the blend. In addition, it may help flow properties and powder compression characteristics. Large granules can be prepared from primary particles by drying from a slurry (with techniques described elsewhere in this text) or by spraying with granulation solution. Figure 13.2(a) shows a top-spray granulator. An alternative method [Figure 13.2(b)] employs an auger to force the blend between rollers, thereby forming a compressed solid that disintegrates into large aggregates (Doelker, 1994).

The steps involved in granulation begin with transferring powders to a mixer and blending the product. The granulation solution can be added, and coarse milling or wet granulation begun. Finally, the product is dried and milled to an appropriate size. If the powder is unstable in the presence of polar solvents, it may be compressed directly. Granulation increases the uniformity of drug distribution in the product, improves the powder flow rate and uniformity of flow, and, if used as an aid to tableting, assists in compression and bonding.

More sophisticated approaches to combining the drug and excipients into a free-flowing large particle size to improve homogeneity, handling, and

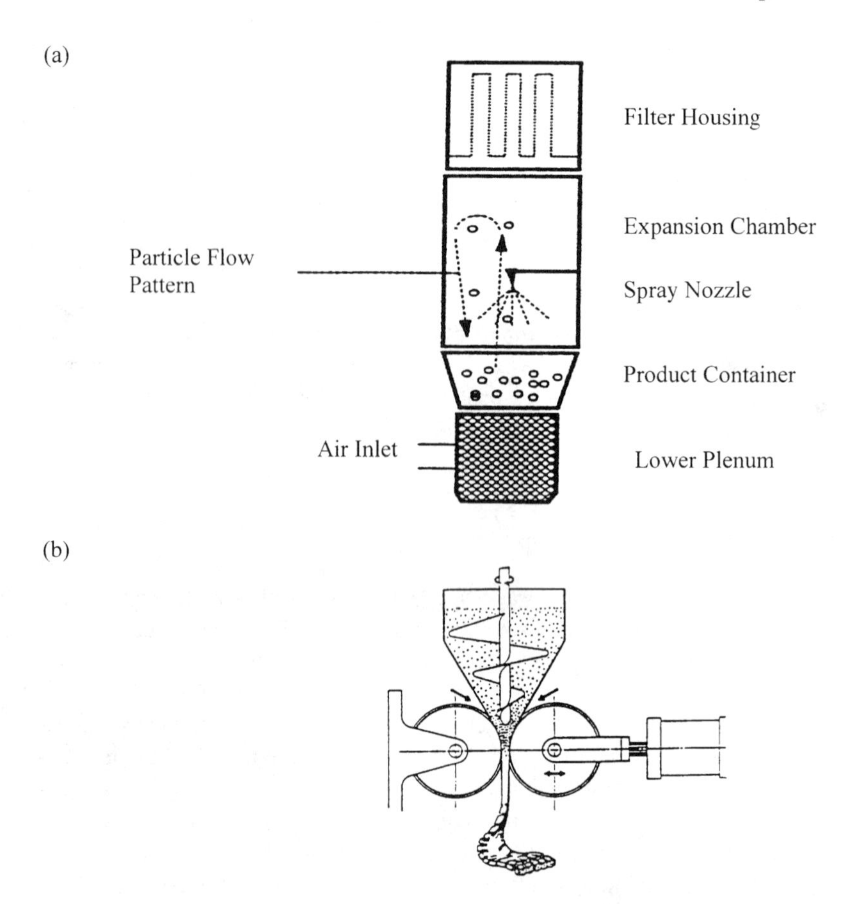


**FIGURE 13.2** (a) Top-spray granulator; (b) granulator with an auger to force the blend between rollers.

drug-release characteristics include spray-drying, fluid-bed-drying, extrusion spheronization, and microsphere or microcapsule formulation. All of these processes are governed to some degree by fundamental fluid flow, heat, and mass transfer phenomena.

## 13.2 HARD CAPSULES

Hard capsules have traditionally been manufactured from gelatin. The gelatin is obtained from bone or skin (calf or pig) acid or alkali treatment over a period of weeks, in some cases as long as 30 weeks (pork skin, 1–5% HCL). The product pH is adjusted, and a hot water extraction is followed by filtration, concentration, and solidification. The final product is milled to size.

Capsule shells are prepared by dipping manganese bronze pins into a bath of molten gelatin. Once removed from the bath the gelatin solidifies on the pins. The caps and bodies are then dried and trimmed. Colorant or titanium dioxide (for opacity) is added as part of this process.

The need for capsules with different physicochemical properties, to aid in stability for example, has promoted a search for alternative materials. In addition, individuals who, for strict religious or health reasons, cannot ingest gelatin need alternative products. In this regard starch and hydroxypropyl-methyl cellulose (HPMC) have been developed. There is no reason to believe that other film-forming polymers might not be useful in this regard. One significant issue that must be considered is the moisture content of the capsule. Gelatin is known to optimally contain 5–15% moisture. Below 5% the shell becomes brittle and may shatter. Above 15% the gelatin distorts, and the shape of dosage form, if not its integrity, is challenged. The presence of a nutrient-rich environment and moisture may offer an ideal situation for microbial growth and enzyme action. Control of microbial growth is therefore a serious consideration in the preparation of capsule products.

Various capsule sizes are manufactured, as shown in Figure 13.3. There are no strict rules for predicting required capsule size. Capsules are selected based on their capacity and the nature of the formulation to be added. The bulk density and compressibility of the product (drug and excipients) dictate the quantity of drug that can be placed within a capsule of known volume. Since the drug dose required to achieve a therapeutic effect can be estimated for new compounds and is known for existing compounds, this information can be used in conjunction with the capsule volume to select an appropriate size.

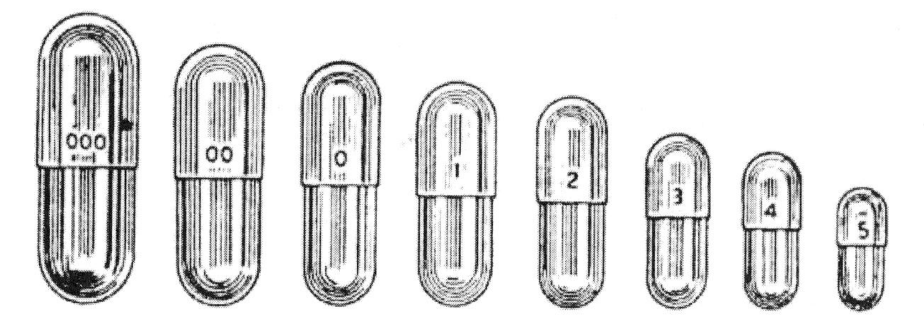


**FIGURE 13.3** Different capsule sizes.

The requirements for capsule production depend on the scale of manufacturing. Extemporaneous preparation (6–12) usually employs enough of the product formula to fill one more capsule than required, to account for loss of fill in manipulation. Special consideration should be given to controlled substances where all of the drug must be accounted for. Industrially (thousands) the amount necessary to fill the desired number can be prepared because the error will be small on such a large scale. The operations involved in large- or small-scale capsule filling are the same. The capsules as supplied in random orientation must be rectified into a bodies-down, caps-up orientation. The two shells are then separated, and the capsule is filled with product formulation. Various methods are available to fill the capsules. For small-scale production, a plate or single capsule filling method is employed. On a larger scale, tamping, intermittent compression, continuous compression vacuum, or auger filling may be employed (Figure 13.4). The shells are then joined and sealed, and the completed product is discharged as shown in Figure 13.5. Different

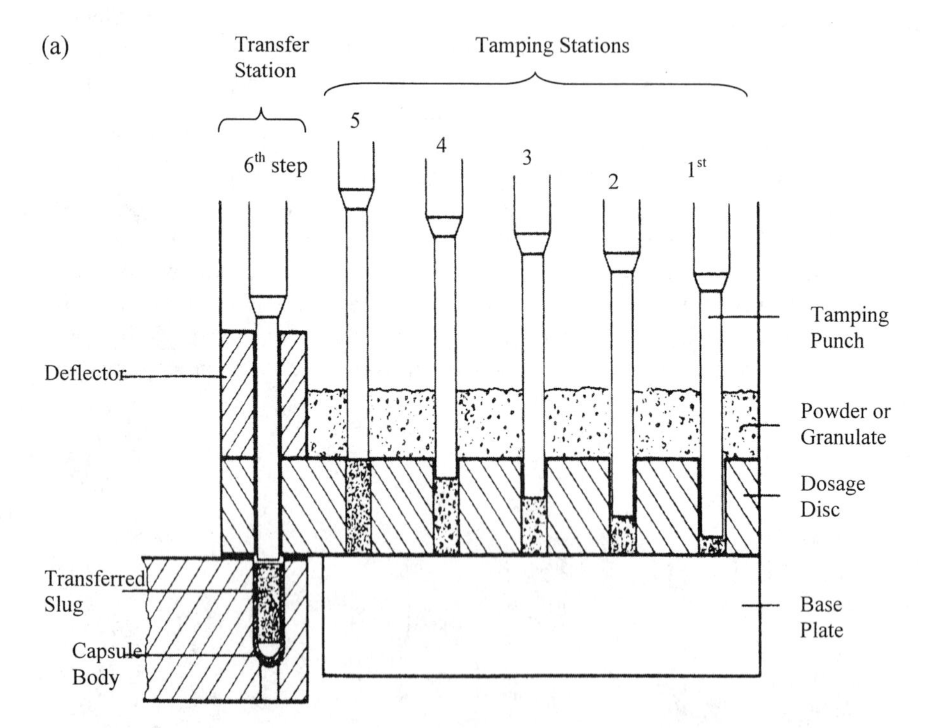


**FIGURE 13.4** Capsule filling: (a) tamping, (b) compression, and (c) auger filling.

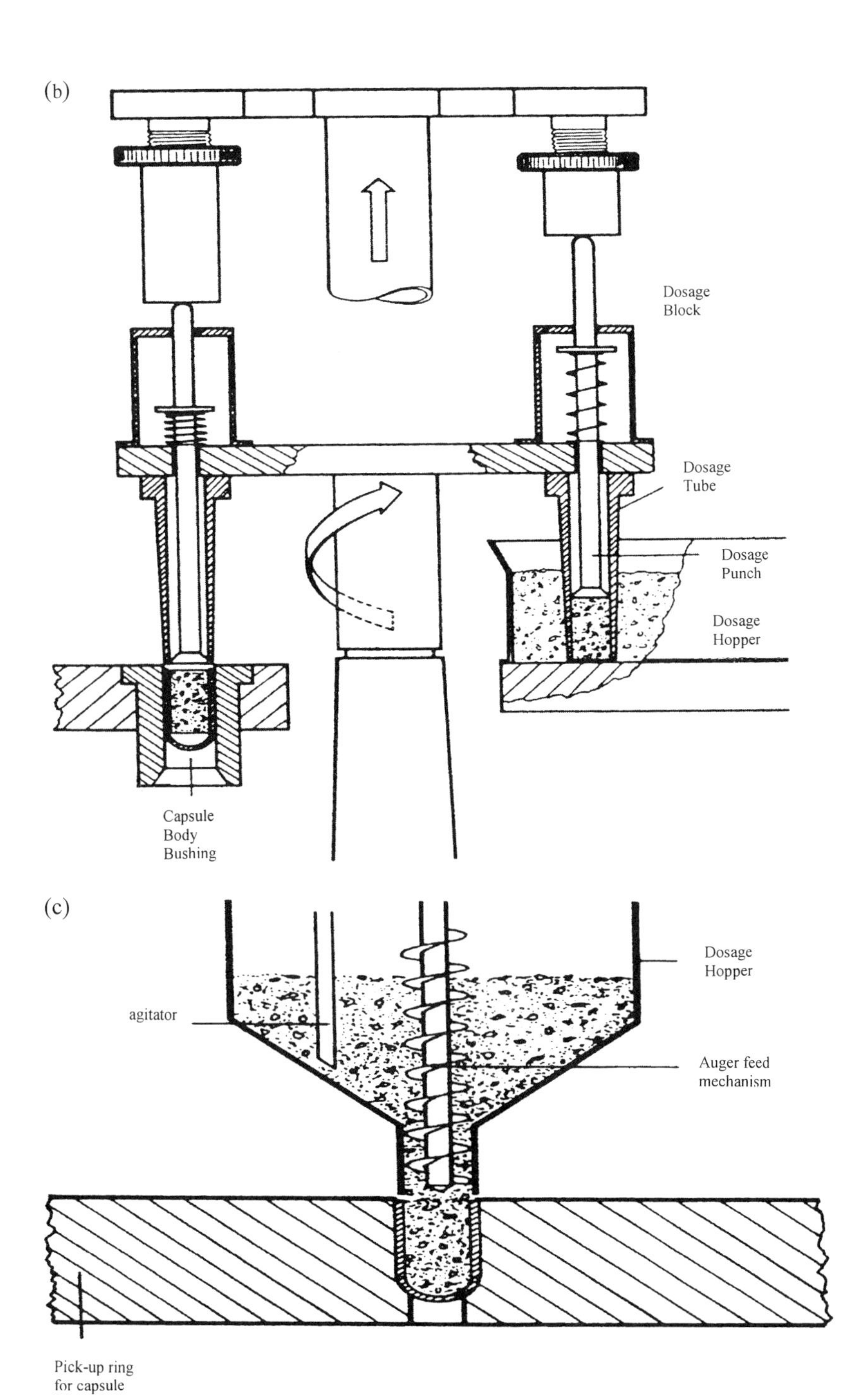

(b)
Dosage
Block
Dosage
Tube
Dosage
Punch
Dosage
Hopper
Capsule
Body
Bushing
(c)
Dosage
Hopper
agitator
Auger feed
mechanism
Pick-up ring
for capsule

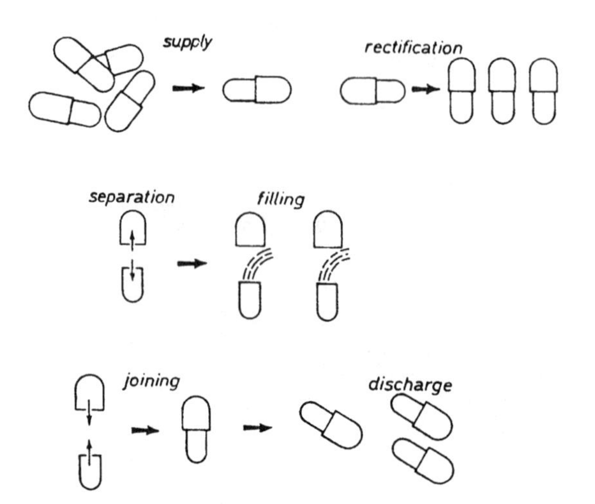


**FIGURE 13.5** Capsule manufacturing process.

locking mechanisms have been developed for capsules shown in Figure 13.6. A cleaning and polishing step also follows the manufacturing procedure to improve product appearance.

The product is visually inspected following production, its potency and uniformity are evaluated, and it is transferred hygienically to the final packaging. If the product is hygroscopic, it may be necessary to package capsules

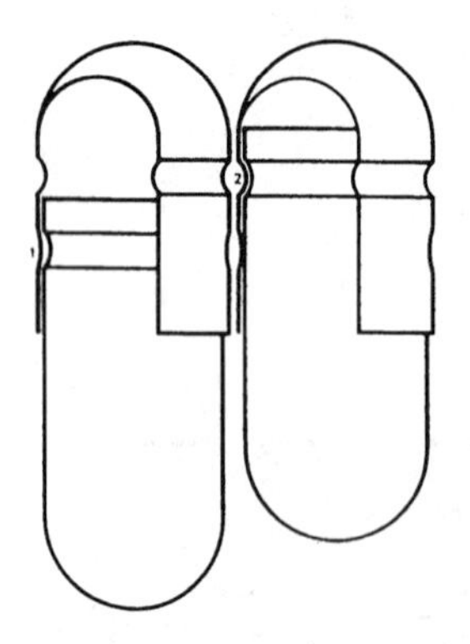

**FIGURE 13.6** Capsule locks.

with desiccant to avoid moisture uptake. Alternatively, impervious packaging materials, such as aluminum blisters, may be used. Capsules are easier to prepare than tablets, are quite flexible with respect to dose, and easily combined with other solid dosage forms since other capsules or tablets can be incorporated into larger capsules.

## 13.3 TABLETS

Additional processes are required for tablet production beyond those described previously. Because these processes are not ubiquitous in pharmaceutical manufacturing, they are dealt with only briefly here. Many of them are required for all solid dosage forms. Each process must be conducted while balancing the effects of the respective excesses.

Compressed solids, tablets, or caplets are prepared by placing the blend of component additives in a cylinder or die, above a movable piston or punch. An upper punch is brought into the top of the piston, and pressure applied to the distal ends of the punches forces the powder into a compact (Figure 13.7). Product quality depends on the cohesive forces acting on the powder under compression. These cohesive forces are influenced by the selection of additives in the dosage formulation. One method of evaluating tablet manufacture considers the effect of applied pressure on porosity of the compressed powder (Carstensen, 1993). Data may be plotted as the negative natural logarithm of porosity against applied pressure in the form of a Heckel plot (Heckel, 1961). The slope is proportional to the yield value ($\phi$, elastic limit) $1/3\phi$.

The tooling of a tablet press varies according to the tablet design. Consideration must be given to the distribution of forces across the faces of the tablet punches as they are brought together to compress the tablet in the die. As more unusually shaped tablets are produced and more elaborate embossing tools are required, the forces are not distributed evenly across the punches, and care must be taken if they are to have a reasonable useful life-span. Mathematically, finite element analysis can be used to characterize these forces and to calculate the requirement for preserving the tools for extended periods.

Coating is achieved by placing a batch of tablets in a coating pan and spraying or coating from solution with the required polymer. The Accela-Cota (Figure 13.8) is one of the more common coating systems.

Tablets have been prepared with different characteristics and for different purposes. The most common tablets are uncoated, coated, chewable, or effervescent. Some specialized dosage forms have been developed for sublin-

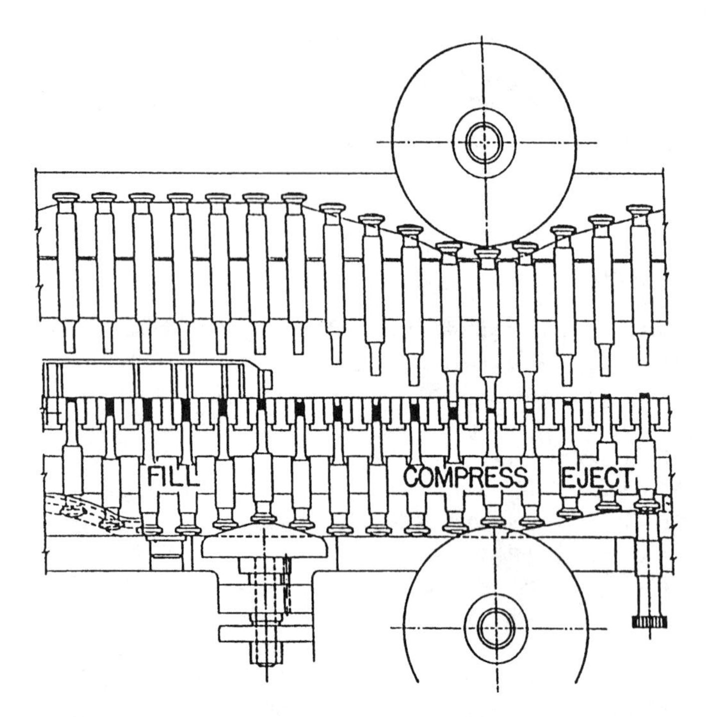


**FIGURE 13.7** Tablet manufacture.

gual and buccal delivery. A typical uncoated conventional tablet might have the composition shown in Table 13.1. Examples of such systems include generic aspirin and Valium. These tablets are designed for rapid dissolution.

Tablets may be coated for a variety of reasons, including better appearance, taste masking, ease of swallowing, protection from light, protection from gastrointestinal irritation, facilitate tablet printing, and control release. The formulation of a coated tablet is similar to an uncoated tablet. Usually it is coated from a solution of polymer, e.g., methylcellulose, enteric polymer. Bayer aspirin or erythromycin products are examples of coated tablets.

Chewable tablets are usually flavored and contain addtives that contribute to a smooth texture, including glycerin and sugars such as mannitol and sorbitol. An example is Tylenol chewable tablets.

Effervescent tablets are formulated such that an acid-base reaction occurs when they are combined with water. This is achieved by using weak acids (e.g., citric, malic, tartaric, or fumeric acids) or bases (e.g., sodium or potas-

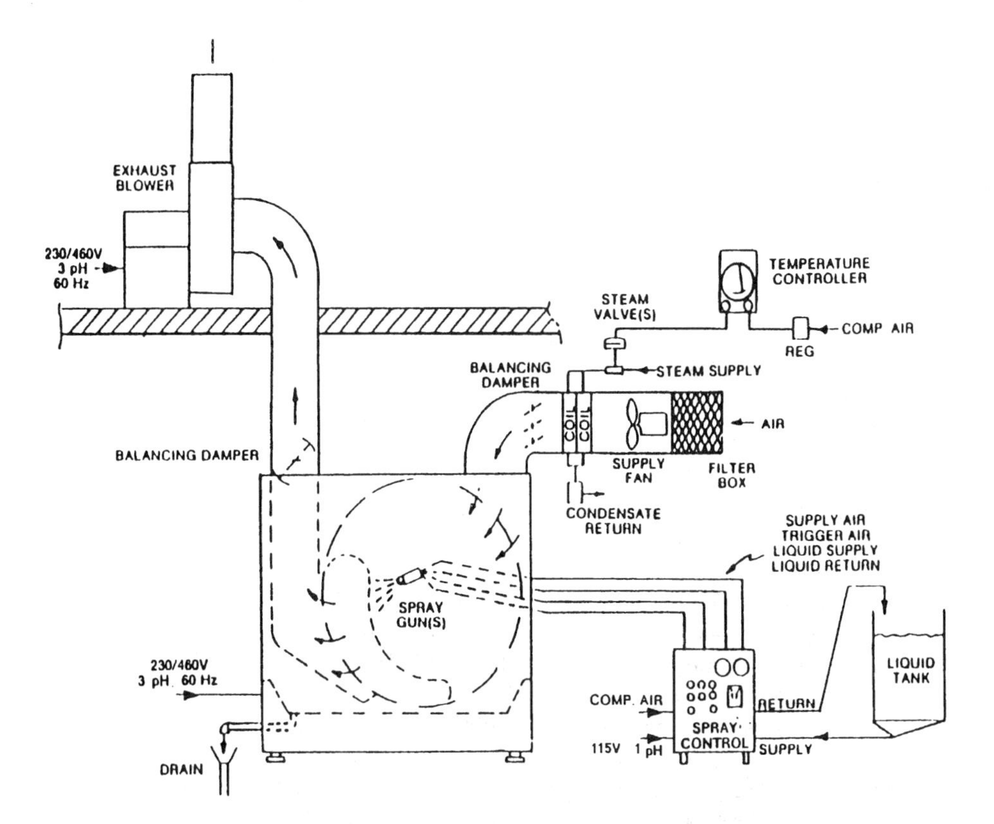


**FIGURE 13.8** Accela-Cota. (Courtesy of Thomas Engineering, Hoffman Estates, Illinois.)

**TABLE 13.1** Tablet Composition

| Purpose | Example |
|---|---|
| Drug | Generic aspirin, Valium |
| Filler | Lactose, sucrose, phosphates |
| Binder | Starch, polyvinylpyrollidone, cellulosics |
| Glidant | Talc, silicon dioxide |
| Lubricant | Magnesium stearate |
| Disintegrant | Starch, sodium starch glycolate |
| Colorant | Various |

sium carbonates) in the product. The best known of these products is Alka-Seltzer.

Sublingual tablets are designed to disintegrate and dissolve instantly. Hence, they must have structural integrity sufficient for storage, transport, and administration but capable of dissolution on the oral mucosa under the tongue. Nitroglycerin tablets designed for treating angina are prepared in a compositionally simple formulation of lactose massed with 60% ethanol. This route of administration is intended to avoid first-pass liver metabolism. Testosterone tablets have been prepared for buccal delivery by slow dissolution. The tablet does not contain a disintegrant and is intended to have an extended residence time in the buccal cavity at the rear of the mouth. Since release is not immediate drug dosage may be significantly reduced by this route.

## 13.4 INHALATION PRODUCTS

Solid particles are employed in two types of inhalation product: the pressurized metered dose inhaler (pMDI) and the dry powder inhaler (DPI). In both cases the method of choice for manufacturing particles in an appropriate size range to deposit in the lungs (<5 μm) is attrition milling by air jet mill.

The pMDI product is prepared as a nonaqueous suspension in which surfactant is used to disperse the drug particles in high-vapor-pressure propellants. Once the particles are prepared the product formulation depends only on the particle dispersion in suspension, their ease of redispersion, and their physical stability upon aerosolization. Figure 13.9 shows a typical filling line for pMDI product.

Dry powder inhaler formulations usually involve a combination of the micronized drug with a carrier, notably lactose. The carrier particles are usu-

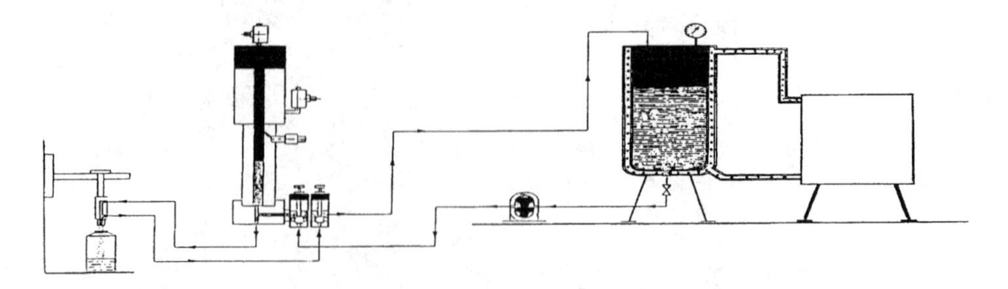

**FIGURE 13.9** Metered dose inhaler filling line.

ally larger than the drug particles and outside the range required for lung deposition (>30 μm). The purpose of these large particles is to help disperse the respirable drug particles carrying them into the inspiratory airflow where they are stripped from the surface as a function of the large shear forces. These formulations are prepared in capsules, blisters, or reservoir devices. The filling technology has been developed to accurately meter small doses into the unit dose packaging.

Other methods of particle preparation have been evaluated, including spray-drying and supercritical fluid manufacture. The capacity to manufacture particles with known and optimized particle size, shape, and surface characteristics is intriguing, and it seems likely that these methods will become more significant in the future and may even surpass micronization for aerosol delivery of drugs.

# 14

# Sterilization

Sterilization processes do not result in a product that can be described as absolutely sterile or nonsterile. The process is a statistical phenomenon. A variety of techniques are available, including heat, radiation, ethylene oxide, and sterile filtration.

## 14.1 THERMAL STERILIZATION

The use of heat to sterilize depends on the magnitude ($T$), duration ($t$), and amount of moisture present:

$$t \propto \frac{1}{T}$$

It is thought that the heat coagulates protein in the living cell. The temperature required for this phenomenon to occur is inversely proportional to moisture present.

### 14.1.1 Dry Heat

Relatively stable substances that resist degradation at high temperatures (>313 K) are suitable candidates for dry heat sterilization. Two hours exposure at 353 K or 45 min at 433 K kills spores as well as vegetative forms of microorganisms. These exposure periods do not include the lag time from loading of the oven until sterilization temperature is achieved. The lag time depends on the geometry and operating features of the oven and characteristics of the load.

The oven types that can be employed are natural and forced convection, both of which are described in Chapter 6. The forced convection oven offers the advantages of uniformity of heat distribution and reduction in lag time in comparison with the natural convection system. This method is reserved almost exclusively for glass or metal, since other materials char (cellulose), oxidize (rubber), or melt (plastic) at these temperatures.

### 14.1.2 Moist Heat

Moist heat offers the advantage of greater effectiveness at low temperatures. The thermal capacity of steam is much greater than that of hot air. Spores and vegetative forms of bacteria may be effectively destroyed in an autoclave employing steam under pressure, either $1.03 \times 10^5$ N/m$^2$ at 394 K for 20 min or $1.86 \times 10^5$ N/m$^2$ at 405 K for 3 min. The lag time to complete exposure of the material to be sterilized is important.

## 14.2 RADIATION

Ultraviolet light is frequently used to reduce airborne microbial contamination and to sterilize surfaces. Both are usually achieved with mercury vapor lamps having an emitted light of $2.537 \times 10^{-7}$ m.

Radiation sterilization uses the ionizing radiation of X-rays and gamma rays. X-rays are derived from bombardment of a heavy-metal target with electrons. Gamma rays are obtained from atomic nucleus decay from the excited state to the ground state.

The energy evolved from radiation can be equated to photon behavior as follows:

$$E = h\nu, \qquad \nu = \frac{C}{\lambda}$$

where $E$ and $\nu$ are the energy and frequency of a photon respectively, $h$ is Planck's constant, and $C$ and $\lambda$ are the speed and wavelength of light, respectively. The energy absorbed from the radiation sources equates to the dose:

$$\begin{aligned} 1 \text{ rad} &= 100 \text{ erg/g of material absorbing} \\ &= 6.24 \times 10^{13} \text{eV/g} \\ &= 2.4 \times 10^{-6} \text{cal/g} \end{aligned}$$

There are a variety of radiation sources. $^{60}$Cobalt ($^{60}$Co) decays to $^{59}$Co in the core of a nuclear reactor to emit two photons ($1.17 \times 10^6$ eV and $1.33 \times 10^6$ eV) and an electron ($0.31 \times 10^6$ eV). The half-time for decay is 5.3 years. $^{137}$Cesium ($^{137}$Cs) decays to emit one photon ($0.661 \times 10^6$ eV). Cesium has a 33-year half-life. An electron beam can be accelerated to an energy equivalent to $5 \times 10^6$–$10 \times 10^6$ eV. At energies below $5 \times 10^6$ eV penetration is insufficient for sterilization. Penetration depth can be correlated with energy levels. For example, materials with density equivalent to water ($\rho = 10^6$ g m$^{-3}$) are penetrated $5 \times 10^7$ m/eV. $^{60}$Co gives rise to radiation that penetrates 0.3 m through water. Accelerating electrons have high dose rate and exposure is only required for seconds. $^{60}$Co has a lower dose rate, so an exposure for hours is required.

Ionizing radiation arises from the photoelectric effect, the Compton effect, or ion pair production. Gamma radiation causes local and intense damage and may break chemical bonds. The primary target is the deoxyribonucleic acid (DNA) of the microorganism. In addition, free radicals may be formed, i.e., peroxides that result in intracellular and extracellular peroxides by a chain reaction, that cause damage.

### 14.2.1 Resistance to Damage

Damage depends on the amount of energy absorbed relative to the number and resistance of the microorganisms being irradiated. Unicellular organisms have greater resistance than multicellular ones. Gram-positive bacteria have greater resistance than Gram-negative bacteria. Finally, bacterial spores have greater resistance than vegetative forms. Viruses are more resistant than bacteria. The energy required to reduce the population of viruses by 90% (Dvalue) is $5 \times 10^5$ rad. Fungi are equivalent to bacterial spores in their resistance.

To evaluate the dose several parameters must be known. What magnitude of source (e.g., $^{60}$Co) is available? A typical source is between $0.5$–$2 \times 10^6$ Curies (Ci), where 1 Ci is $3.7 \times 10^{10}$ disintegrations/s. The product geometry and the speed of the conveyor carrying it to the source must be known.

The dose can be evaluated by a variety of dosimetric techniques. In bulk or ampules containing liquids, ferric ammonium sulfate and ceric sulfate can be used to show an absorbance change, evaluated by UV spectrophotometry. However, this is accurate only for $^{60}Co$ and $^{137}Cs$.

Radiochromic solids can be utilized and evaluated by visible spectrophotometry. Amber and red polymethylmethacrylate are used to evaluate $0.1–1.0 \times 10^6$ or $0.5–5.0 \times 10^6$ rad, respectively. Nylon film is examined for opacity following exposure and may be used to evaluate exposures of $0.1–5.0 \times 10^6$ rad.

Validation requires determination of the bioburden and the Dvalue. These represent the dose required to achieve sterilization and the estimated dose.

The dose may be regarded as overkill if low Dvalues are obtained. *Bacillus pumulis* exhibit inherently high resistance to gamma-ionization radiation with Dvalues of $0.15–0.22 \times 10^6$ rad. The Food and Drug Administration would like a 12-log reduction in microorganisms. The dose required is approximately $2.6 \times 10^6$ rad.

### 14.2.2 Product Development

The product, container, and closure must be evaluated for physical and chemical stability. A number of radiation-induced changes can potentially occur. The product may change in color, odor, flavor, potency, biocompatibility, and toxicity. The container may lose rigidity, become brittle, label adhesion, or become leachable. The product and container may be assessed by exposure to multiple doses and single high doses of radiation. The long-term stability can then be evaluated under ambient storage conditions, at elevated temperatures, and under worst-case shipping conditions.

Dose mapping can be performed by determining the minimum radiation point in the load. Multiple dosimeters can be used to view the vertical quadrant through the load. Dosimeters are routinely set to measure the minimum dose.

## 14.3 ETHYLENE OXIDE

Ethylene oxide is a gaseous alkylating agent used as a surface sterilant. It alkylates proteins, RNA, and DNA in microorganisms, and replaces labile oxygen with ethylene hydroxide. Bulk crystalline materials can occlude vegetative bacterial cells or spores, with crystals. Consequently, ethylene oxide will not reach them. The final step prior to sterilization is aseptic recrystallization.

Ethylene oxide is colorless and aromatic. The threshold limit for the odor is 700 ppm. The OSHA specification for worker exposure is 10 ppm. The toxicity of ethylene oxide is similar to ammonia. It causes conjunctival and respiratory irritation, dizziness, headaches, and vomiting, is known to be mutagenic, and may be carcinogenic. Some by-products of ethylene oxide (bp 283.8 K) are ethylene glycol (bp 471.9 K) and ethylene chlorhydrin (bp 401.4 K). Pure ethylene oxide is flammable and explosive. It is generally mixed with propellant (88:12) or carbon dioxide (90:10). Ethylene oxide polymerizes in the liquid state and may plug lines or spray polymerized sludge on the product. The product expires in 90–120 days because of the polymerization.

Ethylene oxide inactivates all microorganisms. The cidal rate depends on the gas concentration, sterilization temperature, exposure time, and water content of the microorganism. Inactivation follows classical first-order kinetics and is irreversible. Relative humidity is synergistic with ethylene oxide. At 30–60% relative humidity the microorganism hydrates. The water acts as a vehicle to transport the gas through polyethylene and polypropylene. Polystyrene traps ethylene oxide and dissipates it over years and thus is not appropriate for ethylene oxide sterilization. Temperatures of 313–333 K are suitable for heat labile items. Cycle times are longer if temperatures, relative humidities, or ethylene oxide concentrations are lower. Generally, concentrations of 350–700 mg/mL are employed. Cycle times vary from 4–12 hr.

Following sterilization the load is degassed, a dynamic process wherein filtered air is passed over the product for 12–72 hr. Degassing is usually performed in the treatment chamber but may be moved to a sterile facility. The process is monitored with *Bacillus subtilis var. niger* as a biological indicator. Spore strips ($10^6$ spores/strip) can be purchased for this purpose. During validation the load is probed with thermocouples in addition to *B. subtilis* spore strips. Gaseous mixture is sampled from different points in the sterilizer for gas chromatographic analysis.

## 14.4 STERILE FILTRATION

Several filter geometries are available to perform sterile filtration, including flat membranes in a stainless steel press ($<0.293$ m), pleated membranes housed in stainless steel cartridges, and stacked plates in the form of flat segments of membrane filters.

Matrix filters consist of fibers with pores having a depth of up to $1.2 \times 10^{-4}$ m. Cellulose nitrate may be dissolved in the highly volatile solvents amyl acetate, ether, or dioxane. A gel-forming solvent, such as acetone, ethanol, or propanol, may be added. The mixture is poured on a flat plate and placed in a controlled temperature environment to dry. Pore size depends on the gel-forming solvent concentration. Other substances, such as other cellulose esters, acetate, and butyrate, polyamides (nylon), polysulfones, fluorocarbons (Durapore membranes), either polyvinylidenedifluoride (hydrophobic) or surface-modified with organic amides (hydrophilic); acrylic polymers; and polyvinyl chloride, may be used as filter material. To make some membranes hydrophilic surfactants may be added, including Tween 80, Triton X-100, hydroxypropyl cellulose, and glycerol. Sieve filters are made of polycarbonate (Nucleopore $10^{-5}$ m thick). Collimated uranium fission products form nucleation tracks in film. Etching chemical exposure determines pore size.

### 14.4.1 Adsorption and Screening

When wetted almost all membrane filters have negative charge. Bacteria have a similar negative charge and do not necessarily remain on the filter. Filters with other characteristics can be selected under these circumstances. Positively charged (AMF Zeta Plus Membrane) or protein- and peptide-adsorbing (Pall Posidyne Nylon 66) filters can be selected.

Ionic strength, pH, pressure, and flow rate all effect particle adsorption. The flow rate $Q$ through a filter is

$$Q = \frac{\mathrm{Ci}AP}{V}$$

where Ci is the inherent resistance of the filter to flow (a function of void volumes), $A$ is surface area, $P$ is pressure, and $V$ is viscosity.

Filters are related according to nominal pore size and absolute pore size (the largest pore in the filter). Hence, a pore size distribution exists.

### 14.4.2 Filter Integrity

Filter integrity can be evaluated by several techniques. The destructive test involves filtering a suspension of bacterial cells (*Pseudomonas diminuta*, $0.3 \times 10^{-6}$ m) through a $2 \times 10^{-7}$ m filter. Six liters of suspension containing $1 \times 10^{10}$ org/L grow up on an agar plate. Downstream of a $10^{-6}$-m filter there should be nothing and an 8-log reduction should have occurred. The bubble point test, performed before and after sterile filtration, assumes that pores can be characterized as capillaries. When totally wetted all capillaries should be full of water or solution. The pore length is generally much greater than the diameter. Pressure is applied to the wetted filter. The bubble point pressure ($P$) may be described as follows:

$$P = \frac{4\gamma \cos\theta}{D}$$

where $\gamma$ is the surface tension (7.2 $N/m^2$), $\theta$ is the contact angle, and $D$ is the capillary diameter.

### 14.4.3 Product Development Considerations

A specified area of filter must be soaked in a specified volume of product for a designated time. The accelerated stability of a product in the presence of a filter can be performed at 313–333 K for 60 days. The extent of damage, nature and quantity of extractables, and potency of active ingredients must be evaluated prior to selection of a filter for a particular process.

# 15

# Bioprocessing

Bioprocess engineering utilizes microbial growth to produce therapeutic agents of biological origin. In the current climate of recombinant (DNA) technology this often means using host microorganisms as expression vectors for a product, most frequently a protein or peptide.

Many of the principles employed in bioprocess engineering encompass fundamentals and unit processes described elsewhere in the text. All of the fundamentals apply, namely fluid flow and heat and mass transfer. Therefore, unit processes such as pumping (pumps and pipes), sterilization, filtration, heating, and ventilation have an application in bioprocessing. This section covers topics not dealt with earlier: pharmaceutical water systems, bioreactor design, integration and control systems, and product purification.

## 15.1 PHARMACEUTICAL WATER SYSTEMS

In general, pharmaceutical water systems employ combinations of technologies described earlier. However, since the objective is unique, we review some of these methods while introducing issues which are specifically related to the production of different qualities of water (Kuhlman and Coleman, 1991). Table 15.1 summarizes water treatments and uses.

### 15.1.1 Pretreatment and Sources of Water

Potable (drinking) water is not suitable for pharmaceutical purposes. The EPA limits allow 500 recoverable microorganisms per milliliter, none of which can be coliform organisms in drinking water. Drinking water requires further treatment in order to meet the requirements for use in pharmaceutical processes.

Water is pretreated to remove materials likely to be detrimental to the purification equipment. This pretreatment takes many forms. A multimedia bed (different gravels in a carbon steel vessel) is used to remove solids from the municipal water. Common problems include high bacterial or particulate counts in the effluent. This technique is highly inefficient because the container is susceptible to corrosion, the media is porous, and the piping contains dead legs, cracks, and crevices.

### 15.1.2 Water for Injection

Water for injection (WFI) is prepared following pretreatment and further purification, including ion exchange, distillation, and reverse osmosis. WFI must contain 50 recoverable bacterial colonies or less per milliliter for immediate use. Its preparation by distillation or reverse osmosis renders it sterile, from which it must be protected from contamination by endotoxins or microorganisms.

**TABLE 15.1** Water Treatment

| Type of water | Treatment steps |
|---|---|
| Water source (reservoir, ground) | Prefilter, sand, gravel |
| | Zeolite, alum |
| | Filter |
| | Chemical treatment ($Cl^-$, $Fl^-$) |
| Drinking water | Multiple ion exchange (anion, cation) |
| | Charcoal ($Cl^-$, $Fl^-$) |
| | Multiple filters (size discrimination) |
| | Reverse osmosis/distillation |
| WFI | |

*Source*: Modified from Groves (1988).

## Ion Exchange

Zeolite water softener is an exchanger that replaces calcium ions with magnesium ions. Regeneration of the resin is necessary and usually conducted with brine. Consequently, chloride ions which attack certain types of composite membranes may enter the feedwater stream. Bacteria may also propogate in this system.

Activated carbon filters employ a carbon steel tank filled with gravel and covered with activated charcoal (anthracite). Again, this is a source of bacteria and chloride ions.

Deionized water is produced by passing treated water through a mixed bed or a two-bed cation/anion exchange resin system. The resulting water is deionized because hydrogen ions replace cations and hydroxyl ions replace anions. Deionized water has little or no bacteria and is easily regenerated.

The potential for microbial contamination during some of these purification procedures renders additional steps necessary to prepare water suitable for pharmaceutical processing.

## Distillation

Distillation separates water from other soluble and insoluble components by elevating the temperature to that at which vapor forms (100°C) in a boiling chamber and then condensing the vapor into a receiving vessel. The nature of hydrogen bonding of water imparts a unique property to water. Although it can be raised to 100°C with a relatively small amount of energy (80 kcal), it takes almost seven times this amount (540 kcal) to break the hydrogen bonds and release the water as steam at the same temperature. Consequently, in the condensation phase eight times as much water at 5°C (refrigeration temperature) is required to condense the water as steam. These large exchanges of heat may be used in an efficiently designed still to heat up water entering a second still. Alternatively the combined gas law can be utilized by compressing vapor and therefore elevating its temperature (vapor compression still).

## Reverse Osmosis

Reverse osmosis units vary in design, construction materials, and membrane type more than any other unit in the pretreatment process. Usually it is a single-pass system (may not eliminate chlorides). Transmembrane pressures must be maintained. Osmosis is the process whereby a solution separated from pure water by a semipermeable membrane induces movement of water toward the region of high solute concentration. This would ordinarily give rise to an osmotic pressure. If pressure is applied against the osmotic pressure head, the flow of water can be induced in the opposite direction, thereby reversing osmosis. This process, which may be regarded as a form of filtration, removes materials of sizes down to 200 D molecular weight in a sequence that usually removes particulates and viable microorganisms and contaminating molecules sequentially according to size (i.e., large particles, bacteria, viruses, pyrogens, and ions). Softened pH-adjusted water is used to maximize the efficiency of ion removal. The ionic radius affects ions removal, with multivalent ions more readily removed than monovalent ions.

### 15.1.3 Storage and Distribution

The water temperature at the point of use must be such that the water can be handled without risk. A recirculating ambient loop or a heat exchanger at the point of use may be required. A sophisticated system of loops and heat exchangers is required to elevate the water temperature before it returns to a storage tank. One approach is to maintain an ambient loop during the day and heat the water during the night. If the water is maintained at ambient temperatures for not more than 24 hr, the conditions do not violate cGMP regulations.

### 15.1.4 Quality Control

Conductivity and resistivity are convenient on-line measures that ensure water quality. As it circulates, water loses resistivity, stabilizing at about 5 MΩ/cm. Some corrosion may take place in the distribution system, which may ultimately lead to adulteration of the water.

Endotoxin levels are monitored by sampling. Sampled water may be subjected to the limulus amebocyte lysate test to measure the presence of endotoxin. This in vitro assay was predated by rabbit pyrogen testing, which involves monitoring the rabbit's core body temperature in response to injection with a water sample. Endotoxin may cause mild immune responses which will be detected by an increase in body temperature.

### 15.1.5 Validation

Validation of any process is required in pharmaceutical manufacturing. The validation master plan outlines the required content and method of preparing validation documentation. Validation is integral to the start-up of the entire plant. Three major sections of the validation procedure are

1. Installation qualification (IQ): establishes and documents that the unit or system was installed correctly per the manufacturer's specification
2. Operational qualification (OQ): establishes and documents that the unit or system operates as intended
3. Production qualification (PQ): establishes and documents that the unit or system can fulfill its intended purpose on a reproducible basis when challenged with realistic worst-case conditions

The master plan should include a listing of documentation included in validation files for each system (reference files, vendor data, calibration reports, standard operating procedures, and inventories). Critical path schedules, manpower estimates, operator responsibilities, auditing procedures, and outside validation resources should be included in validation documentation.

Outside validation resources should be recruited. They may include purchase of validation protocols from commercial vendors, acquisition of data on validation exercises from equipment vendors, use of testing laboratories for performance qualification, contracting with other qualified agencies to perform water sampling, and, in the extreme case, contract with a qualified agency to perform the entire validation exercise (including writing protocols and performing validation testing). The scale of operation and internal resources dictate which option to select.

## 15.2 CELL KINETICS

### 15.2.1 Definitions

The principles of bioreactor design require understanding the phenomena intended to take place in these controlled environments. This relates to the growth kinetics of prokaryotic or eukaryotic cells derived from animal, plant, or microbial origins. The complexity of biochemical reactions and transport phenomena render accurate predictive mathematical modeling impossible since the system consists of multiple phases having many components. Attempts have been made to estimate growth kinetics based on a matrix combining unstructured or structured approaches to distributed or segregated models (see Table 15.2).

**TABLE 15.2** Various Models for Cell Kinetics

| | Cell components | |
|---|---|---|
| Population | Unstructured | Structured |
| Distributed | Single cells are homogeneously distributed throughout the culture | Cell aggregates are homogeneously distributed throughout the culture |
| Segregated | Single cells are heterogeneously distributed throughout the culture | Cell aggregates are heterogeneously distributed throughout the culture |

*Source*: Modified from Lee (1992).

## 15.2.2 Growth Cycle

The growth cycle of cells has been documented for over a century. It consists of six phases which describe cells growth from an initial period of accommodation or acclimatization through to exhaustion or overpopulation of the environment. The lag phase, which occurs when cells are introduced into a medium, is a period of time when no net change in cell number occurs. This phase is followed by an accelerated growth phase when the cell numbers start to increase and the division rate increases to reach a maximum in the exponential growth phase, where the division rate is proportional to $d \text{ Ln } C_{n0}/dt$, which is constant at maximum value. Following this maximal growth rate a deceleration in both growth and division occurs. The cell population finally reaches a maximum value, but the death of growing cells occurs as nutrients are depleted.

## 15.2.3 Monod Kinetic Parameters

Much has been written regarding the growth of cells in fermenters and chemostats (Lee, 1992). The kinetic considerations in these systems are briefly summarized below.

The Monod equation is an empirical expression describing the effect of substrate concentration on the specific growth rate, and it takes a form similar to Michaelis-Menton enzyme kinetics or the Langmuir adsorption isotherm:

$$\mu = \frac{\mu_{\max} C_s}{K_s + C_s} \tag{15.1}$$

where $\mu$ and $\mu_{max}$ are growth rate and specific growth rate at half-maximum value, and $K_s$ and $C_s$ are a system coefficient and concentration of the limiting substrate in the medium, respectively.

Monod kinetic parameters specific growth rate at half-maximum, and the system coefficient cannot be estimated with a series of individual studies as easily as Michaelis-Menton kinetics for enzyme action. The initial reaction rate can be measured accurately as a function of substrate concentration for enzymes. Cell cultures undergo an initial lag phase in growth in which Monod kinetics do not apply. Even though the Monod equation has the same form as the Michaelis-Menton equation, the rate equation is different.

The Michaelis-Menton equation describing enzyme activity takes the form

$$\frac{dC_p}{dt} = \frac{r_{max} C_s}{K_m + C_s} \tag{15.2}$$

where $C_p$, $C_s$ are product concentration and substrate concentration, respectively, and $K_m$ is the rate constant. The Monod equation takes the form

$$\frac{dC_x}{dt} = \frac{\mu_{max} C_s C_x}{K_m + C_s} \tag{15.3}$$

Note that the cell concentration term $C_x$, in the Monod equation is absent from the Michaelis-Menton equation.

Measuring the steady-state substrate concentration at various flow rates, one can test various kinetic models and estimate the value of the kinetic parameters. A linear relationship can be derived:

$$\frac{1}{\mu} = \frac{K_s}{\mu_{max} C_s} + \frac{1}{\mu_{max}} \tag{15.4}$$

where $\mu$ is equal to the dilution rate ($D$) for a chemostat. If a certain microorganism follows Monod kinetics, the plot of $1/\mu$ versus $1/C_s$ yields the values of $\mu_{max}$ and $K_s$ by reading the intercept and the slope of the straight line. This plot is the same as the Lineweaver-Burk plot for: Michaelis-Menton kinetics. Since $1/\mu$ approaches infinity as the substrate concentration decreases, the data is weighted too heavily at low substrate concentrations and insufficiently at high substrate concentrations. Nevertheless, this approach has the advantage of showing the relationship between the independent ($C_s$) and dependent variables ($\mu$). Figure 15.1 illustrates the manner in which the specific growth rate may be derived from a plot of reciprocal dilution rate versus reciprocal substrate rate.

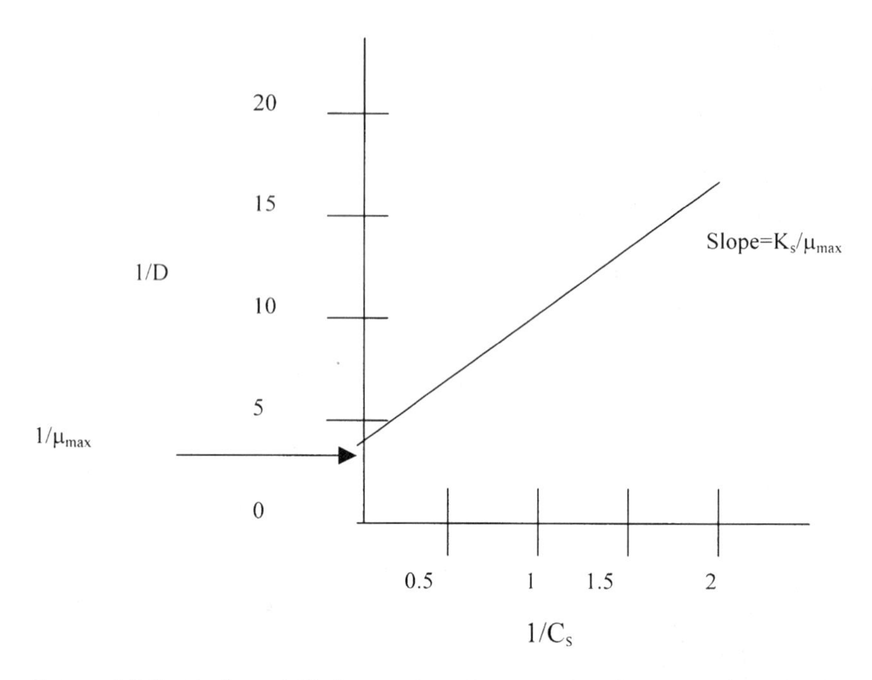


**FIGURE 15.1** Reciprocal dilution rate for a chemostat plotted against reciprocal substrate concentration.

# 15.3 BIOREACTOR DESIGN

## 15.3.1 Background

A bioreactor is a device within which biochemical transformations are caused by the action of enzymes or living cells. The simple method of shaking cells in a flask to enhance oxygenation through the liquid surface and to aid mass transfer of nutrients without cell damage has to be scaled up for industrial processing.

The use of biotechnology in the manufacture of pharmaceuticals is of increasing interest. Consequently, these techniques require attention in the planning of unit processes.

Bioprocessing can be considered in terms of small-scale bioreactors, or fermenters, and the translation of such processes into large-scale economically viable production operations (Klegerman and Groves, 1992; Tatterson, 1994). Bioprocessing is by no means a new field. The topicality of this subject is due to the increasing interest in the use of isolated cells and microorganisms as manufacturing tools. It might well be argued that the technology was developed millenia ago for the purposes of wine and beer production. More recently,

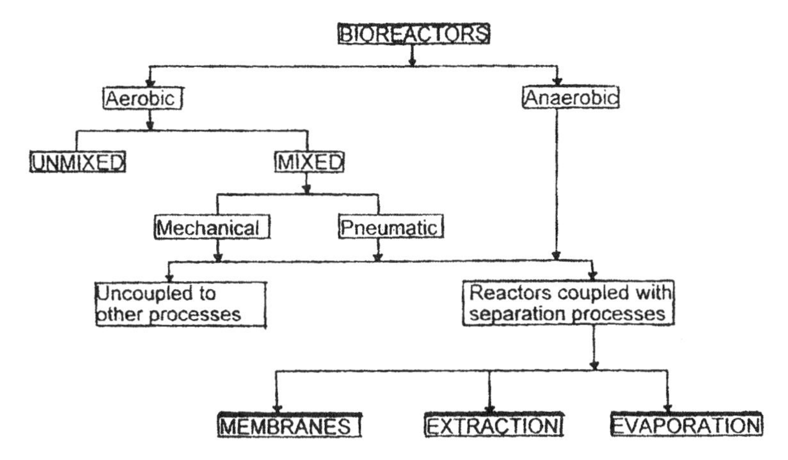


**FIGURE 15.2** Types of bioreactors.

the use of attenuated microorganisms or isolated antigenic materials for vaccination resulted in further developments. In the last decade interest in genetic engineering and manipulation of the genetic code of certain microorganisms has produced a revolution in pharmaceutical manufacturing.

The major difference between a biotechnological process and other pharmaceutical manufacturing operations is the need for a bioreactor (Figure 15.2). A bioreactor may be required to produce expressed proteins utilizing bacteria, yeast, insect, or mammalian cells [ref]. Table 15.3 illustrates the various processes (Prokop and Bajpai, 1991). It would be difficult to describe the various

**TABLE 15.3** Biotechnological Processing

| Stage | Activity | Impact |
|---|---|---|
| First | Reactions: catabolic, anabolic, enzymatic, degradation, and stoichiometric | Molecular |
| Second | Metabolite translocation; compartment differentiation; genetic changes | Individual cells |
| Third | Growth; dispersed, segregated, and mixed culture interactions | Population of cells |
| Fourth | Reaction mixers: mass and heat transfer; dynamics and control; coupled to processes | Bioreactor |
| Fifth | Separation unit operations; process synthesis and integration; quantitative and qualitative evaluation for process design | Process design |

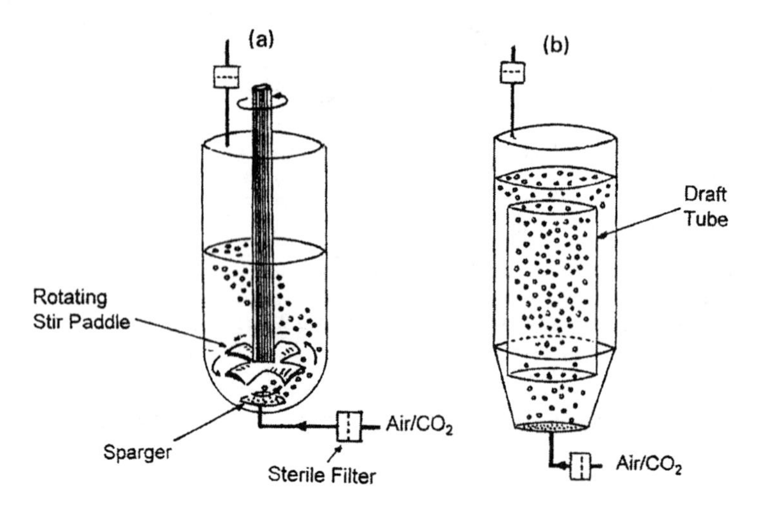


**FIGURE 15.3** Bioreactors: (a) stirred tank reactor; (b) airlift fermenter.

bioreactor elements and their permutations. Some of the simplest examples of bioreactors are shown in Figure 15.3.

Some important factors in bioreactor design are (1) sterility, (2) broth rheology, (3) mass transfer, (4) mixing, (5) heat transfer, (6) suspension homogenization, and (7) shear sensitivity of microorganisms. The importance of these design considerations depends on the nature of the biological systems considered.

## 15.3.2 Rheology

The presence of organized structures in the form of mycelial cells or biopolymers tends to induce non-Newtonian properties in broth. The power law of plastic systems (Martin, 1993) may be employed to describe broth rheology. The viscosity and shear rate are related to the concentration of cell mass in the system. These correlations are species-specific and depend on the stage of growth in the cell cycle.

## 15.3.3 Mass Transfer

Although all nutritient, waste product, and cell integrity issues in growth may be considered in terms of mass transfer, the most notable of these is oxygen transfer for aerobic growth. A maximum uptake rate of oxygen exists for any system, and the design should be based on an understanding of this limitation. Also the oxygen uptake rate of cells shows a saturation dependence on dissolved oxygen concentration. Assuming a pseudo steady state of dissolved oxygen concentration, a design value of gas-liquid mass transfer coefficient $\kappa_L a$ for a biological system can be specified for a specific reactor as

$$\kappa_L a \geq \frac{\text{Maximum oxygen demand}}{C_L^* - C_{L,\text{critical}}}$$

The gas-liquid mass transfer coefficient often changes during the course of fermentation because of changes in broth rheology or through additives, such as antifoaming agents.

### 15.3.4 Mixing

Concentration and temperature are influenced by mixing in bioreactors. Total homogeneity within a system is rarely, if ever, achieved and local variations in mixing within vessels may affect growth, metabolism, or other molecular expression phenomena. Operating conditions influence terminal mixing time (time to reach designated variability associated with complete mixing) and mean circulation time (time to circulate through specific region once). Characterization of mixing times and the influence of geometric features of reactors under different operating conditions and scales of operation (bench, pilot, and full scale) are important if efficiency (time and cost) is to be optimized.

### 15.3.5 Heat Transfer

Heat is dissipated mainly by convection across the walls of the jacket or coils. In aerated systems, metabolic heat production is correlated with oxygen uptake rate. The maximum metabolic load should be considered in design calculations as in gas-liquid oxygen transfer.

Handbook values are available for heat transfer on the jacket side, vessel side, and in tubes. In general, heat transfer becomes a problem only in very large scale operations and in dense microbial populations,which are frequent with recombinant cells. In other cases, gas-liquid mass transfer and mixing are the major concerns.

### 15.3.6 Shear

Agitation is required to maintain suspensions of the cells. Agitated bioreactors are designed to maintain complete suspension (no cell mass at the bottom of the reactor) or a homogeneous suspension. These terms imply stable flocculations (aggregates) in suspension or homogeneous cell distribution throughout the suspension.

The mechanism of shear damage to the cells is not clear. Mycelial or protozoan cells exhibit shear-rate-limited growth, and cell damage has been monitored by analyzing the concentration of low-molecular-weight nucleotides in the culture broth.

## 15.4 BIOPROCESSING PLANT DESIGN

The foregoing discussion focused on major elements of bioprocessing activities, namely water treatment and reactor design. Heating, ventilation, and air conditioning (HVAC) and steam production, described elsewhere in this text, are also requirements for bioprocessing. The design of a bioprocessing plant is subject to current good manufacturing practices (cGMPs), which emphasize control and reproducibility. It is clear that the application of such principles to other pharmaceutical processes of a more mechanical nature may readily be achieved. The biological nature of the processes being controlled challenges the engineers and scientists involved.

As with any regulated process specifications must be prepared in advance and acceptance criteria established for subsequent quality control checks. Validation of the facility and process should be considered essential to design, construction, and start-up. Documentation of design and construction ensures appropriate specifications for subsequent validation.

## 15.5 PROTEIN PURIFICATION

The purpose of bioprocess engineering is to utilize resources necessary to promote the growth of microorganisms in a controlled environment for the purpose of producing a product of biological origin. Note that additional processing is required to purify the product obtained from these systems. The purification from cell culture of soluble proteins may be conducted by combining traditional purification steps (Harrison, 1994). These steps are shown in Table 15.4. Each step focuses on particular physicochemical properties; for

**Table 15.4** Purification Steps of Soluble Proteins

| | |
|---|---|
| Chromatography | Adsorption Ion exchange (IEC) Hydrophobic interaction (HIC) Gel Affinity High-pressure liquid chromatography (HPLC) |
| Precipitation | Ammonium sulfate |
| | Organic solvents |
| | High-molecular-weight polymers |
| Extraction | Liquid-liquid |
| | Solid-liquid |
| Concentration | Ultrafiltration |
| Buffer exchange | Ultrafiltration |
| | Gel chromatography |

example, ion exchange, hydrophobic interaction, and gel chromatography separate molecules based on charge, hydrophobicity, and molecular size, respectively. Inclusion bodies with complex tertiary structures undergo additional steps, including washing, solubilizing, and refolding of proteins before further purification steps are adopted.

As with all of the foregoing processes, validation of purification steps is required. Indeed, the sequence of designing protein purification processes may be described as follows (Nelson, 1991):

- Stepwise recovery yields
- Impurity removal
- Scalability of protein purification steps
- Validation of protein purification steps

Biotechnological innovation occurs as the result of complex integrated bioprocesses based on molecular and cellular biology. The key processes have been described briefly in this chapter, and discourses of some length are available on each of these topics in the literature. Since the next generation of pharmaceutical products is likely to be developed by these methods, readers are strongly encouraged to familiarize themselves with these topics and with the more fundamental issues of molecular and cellular biology not covered in this text (Bolsover et al., 1997).

# References

Bolsover SR, Hyams JS, Jones S, Shephard EA, White HA. From Genes to Cells. New York: Wiley, 1997.
Carstensen JT. Pharmaceutical Principles of Solid Dosage Forms. Lancaster, PA: Technomic, 1993, p. 73.
Crowder TM, Hickey AJ. The physics of powder flow applied to pharmaceutical solids. Pharm Tech Feb. 50–58, 2000.
Doelker E. In: Chulia D, Deleuil M, Pourcelot Y, eds. Powder Technology and Pharmaceutical Processes. Amsterdam: Elsevier, pp. 403–471, 1994.
Dushman S, Lafferty JM. Scientific Foundations of Vacuum Technique. 2nd ed. New York: Wiley, 1962, p. 48.
Fung HL. In: Banker GS, Rhodes CT, eds. Modern Pharmaceutics. New York: Marcel Dekker, 1990, pp. 209–237.
Gammage RD, Glasson DR. Chemistry and Industry 1963, p. 1466.
Gregg SJ. Trans Br Ceram Soc 54: 257, 1995.
Groves MJ. Parenteral Technology Manual. 2nd ed. Buffalo Grove, IL: Interpharm Press, 1988, pp. 17–36.
Harrison RG. Protein Purification Process Engineering. New York: Marcel Dekker, 1994.
Heckel RW. Trans Metal Soc AIME 221: 671 (1961).

Heywood H. In: Cremer HW, Davies T, eds. Chemical Engineering Practice. Butterworths, 3: 8, 1957.
Hickey AJ. Lung deposition and clearance of pharmaceutical aerosols: What can be learned from inhalation toxicology an industrial hygiene. Aerosol Sci Tech 18: 290–304, 1993.
Hinds WC. Aerosols Technology, Properties Behavior and Measurement of Airborne Particles. New York: Wiley, 1982, pp. 164–186.
Jennings TA. J Parent Sci Tech 42: 118–121, 1988.
Klegerman ME, Groves MJ. In: Pringle AT, ed. Pharmaceutical Biotechnology: Fundamentals and Essentials. Buffalo Grove, IL: Interpharm Press, 1992, pp. 115–137.
Kuhlman H, Coleman D. In: Avis KE, ed. Process Engineering Applications. Buffalo Grove, IL: Interpharm Press, 1995, pp. 221–268.
Lacey PMC. Trans Instn Chem Engrs 21: 53, 1953.
Lee JM. Biochemical Engineering. Englewood Cliffs, NJ: Prentice Hall. 1992, pp. 138–189.
Martin A. Physical Pharmacy. 4th ed. Baltimore: Williams & Wilkins, 1993, pp. 212–251.
Masters K. Spray Drying Handbook. New York: Langman Scientific & Technical, 1991.
McCabe WL, Smith JC, and Harriott P. Unit Operations of Chemical Engineering. 5th ed. New York: McGraw Hill, 1993.
Mullin JW. Crystallization. 3rd ed. New York: Butterworth-Heinemann, 1993, pp. 1–28.
Nail SN. J Parent Drug Assoc 34: 358–368, 1980.
Nelson KL. In: Prokop A, Bajpai RK, Ho C, eds. Recombinant DNA Technology and Applications. New York: McGraw-Hill, 1991, pp. 415–459.
Newman ACC, Axon A. Soc Chem Ind Monograph No. 14: 291, 1961.
Perry RH, Chilton CH. Chemical Engineers' Handbook. 5th ed. New York: McGraw-Hill, 1973.
Pikal MJ, Roy ML, Shah S. J Pharm Sci 73: 1224–1237, 1984.
Pillai RS, Yeates DB, Miller IF, Hickey AJ. Controlled release from condensation coated respirable aerosol particles. J Aerosol Sci 25: 461–477, 1993.
Prokop A, Bajpai RK. In: Prokop A, Bajpai RK, Ho C, eds. Recombinant DNA Technology and Applications. New York: McGraw-Hill, 1991, pp. 415–459.
Sacchetti M, Van Oort M. In: Hickey AJ, ed. Inhalation Aerosols. New York: Marcel Dekker, 1996, pp. 337–384.
Tatterson GB. Scaleup and Design of Industrial Mixing Processes. New York: McGraw-Hill, 1994.
Thompson SK. Sampling. New York: Wiley, 1992.
Train D. Pharm J 185: 129, 1960.
Wagner JG, J Pharm Sci 50: 359, 1961.

# Bibliography

Allen T, Particle Size Measurement. 4th ed. New York: Chapman and Hall, 1990.
Andrews GA, Kniseley RM, Wagner HN. Radioactive Pharmaceuticals. US Atomic Energy Commission, 1996.
Ansel HC, Popovich NG, Allen L. 6th ed. Pharmaceutical Dosage Forms and Drug Delivery Systems, Malvern, PA: Williams and Wilkins, 1995.
Beard J. Dynamics of Fluids in Porous Media. Mineola, NY: Dover, 1972.
Bird RB, Stewart WE, Lightfoot EN. Transport Phenomena, New York: Wiley, 1960.
Carey VP. Liquid-Vapor Phase-Change Phenomena. New York: Hemisphere, 1992.
Cheremisinoff NP, ed. Air/Particulate Instrumentation and Analysis. Ann Arbor, MI: Ann Arbor Science, 1981.
Cheremisinoff NP. Practical Fluid Mechanics for Engineers and Scientists. Lancaster, PA: Technomic 1990.
Chhabra RP. Bubbles, Drops and Particles in Non-Newtonian Fluids. Boca Raton, FL: CRC Press, 1993.
Cho YI, Hartnett JP. Advances in heat transfer. 15:59–141, 1982. Non-Newtonian fluids in circular pipe flow.
Chulia D, Deleuil M, Pourelot Y. Powder Technology and Pharmaceutical Processes. Amsterdam: Elsevier Science, 1994.

Coulson JM, Richardson JF. Chemical Engineering. Vol 1, 3rd ed. New York: Pergamon Press, 1977.
Crank J. The Mathematics of Diffusion. 2nd ed. Oxford, UK: Oxford University Clarendon Press, 1975 (reprinted 1992).
Cussler EL. Diffusion Mass Transfer in Fluid Systems. New York: Cambridge University Press, 1984.
Fayed ME, Otten L, eds. Handbook of Powder Science and Technology. New York: Van Nostrand Reinhold, 1984.
Groves MJ, Olson WP, Anisfield MH. Sterile Pharmaceutical Manufacturing. Buffalo Grove, IL: Interpharm Press, 1991.
Hartnett JP, Kostic M. Advances in Heat Transfer 19:247–356, 1989. Heat transfer to Newtonian and non-Newtonian fluids in rectangular ducts.
Hesketh HE, El-Shobosky MS. Predicting and Measuring Fugitive Dust. Lancaster, PA: Technomic, 1985.
Hyman D. Mixing and agitation. In: Advances in Chemical Engineering. Vol. 3. Academic Press, 1962.
Lachman L, Lieberman HA, Kanig JL. The Theory and Practice of Industrial Pharmacy. 3rd ed. Philadelphia: Lea and Febiger, 1986.
Lefebvre AH. Atomization and Sprays. New York: Hemisphere, 1989.
Little A, Mitchell KA. Tablet Making. 2nd ed. Liverpool: Northern, 1963.
Meyer RE. Introduction to Mathematical Fluid Dynamics. Mineola, NY: Dover, 1982.
Neumann BS. The flow properties of powders. In: Advances in Pharmaceutical Sciences, Vol. 2. New York: Academic Press, 1967, pp. 181–221.
Orr C. Particulate Technology. New York: Macmillan, 1966.
Ozisik MN. Boundary Value Problems of Heat Conduction. Mineola, NY: Dover, 1968.
Pietsch W. Size Enlargement by Agglomeration. New York: Wiley, 1991.
Prandtl L, Tietjens OG. Fundamentals of Hydro- and Aeromechanics. Mineola, NY: Dover, 1957.
Rietema K. The Dynamics of Fine Powders. New York: Elsevier, 1991.
Rumpf H. Particle Technology. London: Chapman and Hall, 1990.
Taylor R, Krishna R. Multicomponent Mass Transfer. New York: Wiley, 1993.
Tien C. Granulator Filtration of Aerosols and Hydrosols. Boston: Butterworths, 1989.
Van-Hook A. Crystallization: Theory and Practice. ACS. Monograph No. 152, London: Chapman and Hall, 1961.
Weidenbaum SS. Mixing of solids. In: Advances in Chemical Engineering. Vol. 2. Academic Press, 1958.
Wert CA, Thomson RM. The Physics of Solids. 2nd ed. New York: McGraw-Hill, 1970.

# Index